Unaltered

A New Perspective

Donna Lammar

MEDICAL AND GENERAL DISCLAIMER FOR UNALTERED

Find Donna & Beautifully Unprocessed online:
Facebook:
https://www.facebook.com/beautifullyunprocessed
Website: http://beautifullyunprocessed.blogspot.com/
Twitter: https://twitter.com/BUnprocessed

Find more ways to connect on the website…

DEDICATION

To my amazing, faithful, and absolutely loving husband, to our three precious daughters, who always encourage me to keep trying.

Thank you for your faithful love, encouragement, prayer, and support. You are truly blessings from God.

To my husband grandmother Marjean, thank you for inspiring me these past thirteen plus years. To extended family who've supported me with ideas, inspiration, and guidance.

To my prayer warriors, your fervent prayers gave me the extra oomph I needed during times of trial. I truly appreciate your dedication.

Thank you to two amazing strong Godly women Cora and Diane you guided me through this journey, empowered me with your words, helped me become more educated and inspired me from the start.

To my supportive friend Sarah, thank you for your positive encouragement, late night chats, and advice. There were moments I just felt stuck, you shared your kind words and inspired me to just stay real to myself and family.

Most importantly, to our heavenly Father, who has given me and my family the strength and power to push on when the world is against us.

CONTENTS

INTRODUCTION

This book is about our journey. It's been filled with tears, joy, laughter and more. We've had to change our lives to save our daughter from seizures and other health problems.

Because of the changes we had to make to our lives we've not only become healthier while doing it but smarter in the process.

We've had to turn our back on the worldly view we once had, open our hearts to God, and trust in the unseen.

So now the time has come that I've been led to share our story and reach out by writing this book. I want to bring awareness to other parents who feel lost, desperate, and are tired of fighting for what seems to be an endless battle filled with sleepless nights.

You may be reading this because it's you who is struggling with illness; you've gotten tired of not having answers, either way, no matter what the circumstance I hope you'll find some answers.

In the book I will touch on how to encourage change within your lifestyle and ways to build your health, and how to make your own healthier (non-toxic) cleaners right in the comfort of your own home.

You'll find that there may be parts of the book that seem tedious, boring, or just lacking in pizzazz (there aren't too many) just remember, to really get the full benefits you'll need to keep focused and read on. It will be worth it!

You'll find that I've included a nice assortment of information about these things that can harm you and your precious family as well as alternatives that are safer for you and your family.

Instead of always running to the doctor's office or running to the medicine cabinet, read my book and see how you can help heal your body.

Take the step to live an unaltered life. This doesn't mean cutting off your entire life to the world like you may think, so don't go into a panic.

You'll find yourself learning about the remedies and medicines of the past our parents, grandparents, and great grandparents used. Learn how the old ways were so much healthier and
unaltered.

I'm no doctor; I'm just a mom who wanted better for my children. I chose to give up the control I thought I had, took a deep breath, dropped to my knees and begged God to lead us in the right direction to heal our daughter and life.

Yes, I did say the "G" word God, please don't go into a panic, weather you follow Christ or not I welcome you with open arms to read this book. It's designed for everyone and anyone who wants to take the step to living unaltered and healthier.

 I want to help you take that step; if you have questions please I beg of you, take a moment and contact me. I'm available on my blog, fb, and by email.

So please take the time to read my book, and take the step to a better unaltered version of life.

God bless,
Donna Lammar
Author & Blogger at Beautifully Unprocessed

Unaltered

1

THIS IS OUR LIFE,
JUST THE BASICS

~

"HE WILL WIPE EVERY TEAR FROM THEIR EYES.
THEREW ILL BE NO MORE DEATH' OR MOURNING
OR CRYING OR PAIN, FOR THE OLD ORDER OF
HTINGS HAS PASSED AWAY."
-REVELATION 21:4 NIV

This is where our journey begins. Our journey has brought us closer to God, however further away from the world. You may wonder what exactly that means, don't for a minute think we took a leap onto the crazy train and secluded our children from the world because that's not at all what I'm saying.

In 2006 we were blessed with a beautiful 9lb 15oz little girl. We felt so blessed, and then it all began. Our precious little girl turned purple. I looked to the nurse as she was wheeling us to our room, I told her our baby was turning purple. She tried to reassure me that it's normal, I scolded her and said "NO this is not normal she is PURPLE!"

She suddenly looked and panicked as she realized this precious new baby was indeed turning purple. From head to toe my baby was purple. The valve in her heart had not closed completely. Suddenly doctors and nurses grabbed her and ran off, I was so scared and all I could do was hope she'd be okay. I didn't know God all that well at the time so I depended on my husband to make everything okay. However, I know that God was with us the whole time and he watched over our precious baby.

We waited and waited and waited some more, until finally a doctor came to our room and informed us of her condition. He told us she would be kept for observation in the NICU for a few hours. Finally she was brought to me. I was so thankful to hold her once again.

However, only to realize that every time we would hold her, her limbs would become purple. The doctors told us there was nothing they were able to do for us. We were scared and helpless with no options to help her.

The doctors had given us nothing, no hope at all. As parents of a new baby we were frustrated, angry, scared, and not sure what we were supposed to do for this precious new little girl.

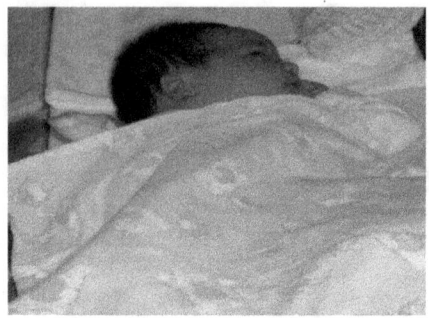

(Pumpkin at the hospital)

After a few days we were able to return to home. We had no idea what would follow and that our adventure had not even began yet. Not only did we have a new born with heart issues and well even more to come, we also had a two and a half year old little girl who would become extremely rebellious over the next couple of months.

To make the first part of our adventure short, otherwise it would take up the whole book; I'll share some tidbits.

Our newborn had severe colic, which meant endless nights of crying both from her and mommy. My husband was working two jobs, so he couldn't help as much as he wanted. I was and still am thankful for all he did though.

The 2 ½ year old would wake from all the crying, so mommy would cry even more. For the first year, one to two hours of sleep is what this stressed out, strung out, exhausted mommy would get for sleep.

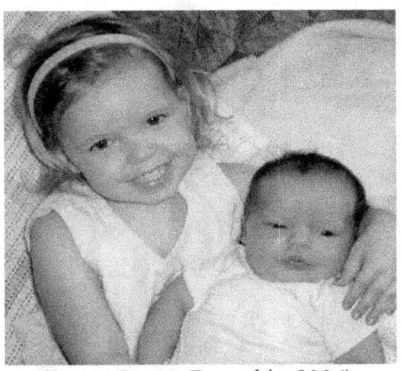

(Sweet Pea & Pumpkin 2006)

After she grew out of her colic, we started attending church and fell in love with our glorious amazing Lord. Let me tell you without him, there is no way we would have been able to handle the next part of the journey.

Over the next couple of years everything seemed to be great, her heart had finally healed correctly and she was a happy kid. We had another beautiful little girl sugar and life seemed wonderful.

However, when she turned five our world was suddenly turned upside down and twirled around like a roller coaster. We were devastated, we were lost, and had absolutely no control or so we thought.

My little pumpkin, now being five was having seizures, seizures of all things. Every night it seemed to occur, she'd go to sleep with everything being just fine, she'd be happy and content, and then suddenly would wake with these horrifying screams. She never seemed to know what was going on, she'd shake uncontrollably and her eyes would roll into the back of her head.

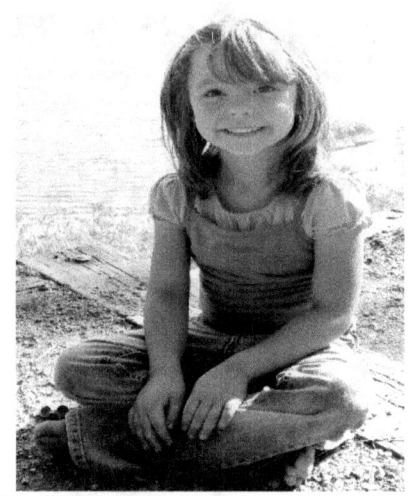

(Pumpkin age 5 enjoying a day out 2011)

I had called the nurse hot-line so many times and they just told me to hold her, there was nothing they could do. I remember holding her in my arms and just crying my eyes out, begging God to let her be okay. "Give her another day Lord", I'd beg. I'd pray and beg him no matter how long the seizure was, I'd just beg and pray that she'd be okay.

We started taking her to doctor after doctor, we traveled out of state to try to find new doctors, none, not one had an answer.

They threw labels such as ADD, ADHD, Autism, ODD, and many others at us. We were so overwhelmed with all the nonsense and lack of answers.

We prayed and prayed and prayed that God would give us answers because all these doctors finally admitted they didn't know what was causing the problems. The seizures were unexplained and the only answer they had was medicine that would affect her heart, and had no guarantee of getting rid of the seizures.

I was so angry, I found myself getting angry with God because he was letting this happen, why would he let this precious five year old little girl go through this. Did I do something wrong? Was I the reason she was suffering?

I then felt God push me in the right direction; it wasn't doctors we needed or medicines. It was a change in our lifestyle.

That's where the journey got very interesting. We'd find that the things we used on a daily basis would either cause her to have a seizure, or would cause her not to have one at all.

It was a tremendous breakthrough for our family; however it took us about a year to really figure it out.

To keep it this short, we found out our daughter is allergic to artificial dyes, artificial fragrances, most pesticides, and has sensitivity to gluten.

This may not seem all that horrible to someone who hasn't had to base their lives around not having these things. However, I'm pretty sure that's why God led our family through this, and why he has led me to write this book.

Our world is over consumed with all this junk and more! I'd like to challenge you to go to the grocery store and explore, explore through the aisles and see how many dyes are in the daily things you use. It's truly absurd how many of our day to day items are filled with artificial junk!

Share your experiences with us; tell us how many items you found in your local grocery market. Share your feeling with us. We'd love to hear your thoughts.

So with all the sadness and turmoil of our journey, let me share the amazing part. Not only did we grow closer to God, our marriage has grown stronger, we've grown into better parents, and to make it all worthwhile…

Our precious Pumpkin has now been seizure free for two years and counting! Her anniversary date for being seizure free is July 12th.

She loves counting down the days when it's coming close so she can say how long it's been that she's been seizure free.

This was not by the help of doctors, but from trusting in God, changing our life style, how we eat, what products we use in our home, etc.

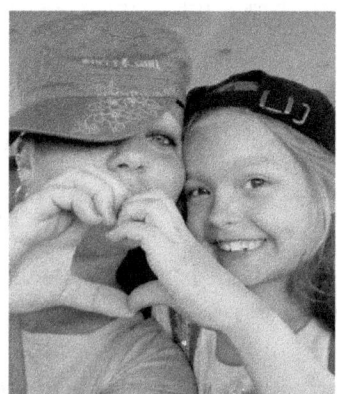

(Mommy & Pumpkin being silly 2014)

Life has continued to have its bumps and at times even what seemed like mountains to us. However we've pushed on, held strong to our faith and trusted that everything would work out as it should.

Pumpkin will be nine come June; she still has some special areas in her life which we don't label anymore. Instead we call them her gifts. This is where we move on to the next part of our journey, day to day life.

We homeschool our three daughters and to be honest I personally love it as it gives me time to really get to know each of them on a very real level. Instead of the world shaping my children, I get to watch God shape them and watch their beautiful personalities bloom.

Pumpkin, Sweet Pea, and Sugar are so much alike yet at the same time are very much different. There are days they get along great and hang out, then there are those days that Pumpkin just can't handle the chaos and noise.

We eat real food, don't worry we don't eat some powdered stuff or anything weird. Well unless you want to call our girls weird because they'd rather have fruit and veggies over candy most days. That is kind of weird; however you won't find this mama complaining.

You can often find us playing, learning, or exploring. This journey is far from over I'm sure, with God's grace we hope to one day reach out further and make a difference in the world.

Pumpkin has even written a letter to Mrs. Obama, she hopes that it will bring awareness and maybe just maybe a change.

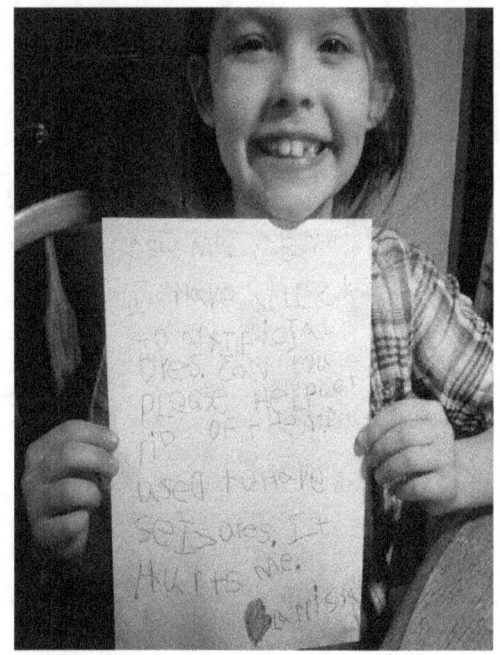

(Pumpkin & her letter to Mrs. Obama '15)
So let's move on.. To the hard stuff.

2

INFLUENCE BEYOND MEASURE,
THEY DON'T WANT YOU TO KNOW.

~

"DO NOT BE MISLED, BAD COMPANY CORUPTS
GOOD CHARACTER."
-1 CORINTHIANS 15:33A

Colorants & Artificial Dyes

Before you get started with this chapter let me tell you ahead of time it will be the hardest to get through. It can be boring yet intriguing, please don't pass it by. It will be worth it.

The information is genuine and it will teach you more than you can probably imagine. I've learned a lot through this journey and hope that it helps you as much as it's helped our family.

Keeping everything perfect in life and in your home is generally impossible, that is unless you live in a pretend world. Which unfortunately most people are and just don't realize it. Now you're probably wondering what in the world I'm talking about.

Well if you knew what was in your favorite shampoo or favorite cleaner and what it's really doing to your family, you'd realize you've been living in a world of pretend.

If you just grab something off the shelf, or even if you've done lots of reviewing to see how great these products are, unfortunately you've probably been lied to, stolen from, and well straight out deceived by the large companies that your purchasing from.

Before our daughter was born I had no problem at all using regular cleaners from the store, bath and body products, laundry detergents of all sorts and all the basic stuff you probably use every single day in your own home. However, that changed quite rapidly and unexpectedly for our family.

After our daughter was born things changed for us. As time went on with her we couldn't just use whatever we wanted to. She started having seizures, outbreaks of hives, headaches, rashes, pains all over her body, and tantrums like

I'd never seen before out of any child.

To be quite honest there were times when I questioned my own sanity because of the restless days that never seemed to end, the nights of crying and uncontrollable tantrums. I questioned if I was being a good enough mom, if I was making my child suffer somehow, if maybe I was the reason that my daughter was behaving like this. I couldn't understand what was happening or why in the world it was.

After we had talked with local doctors went to doctor after doctor and were left with no answers. We traveled out of state and paid out of pocket to see specialists, who had no answers for us which led us to paying thousands of dollars out of our pocket because the insurance didn't want to cover the medical bills anymore.

We talked to friends, family, teachers, and other people who maybe would have some sort of idea of what was going on with our precious little girl.

At only five years of age, she was extremely abusive when she'd have tantrums. These tantrums were so out of control it would result in bruises, bloody noses, scratches, scrapes, holes in the walls, etc. She was not only abusive to herself by anyone that came within her reach while she was having one.

As if this wasn't enough to already handle then she'd break out in some sort of rash or hives almost every time she'd eat. We couldn't understand what in the world was going on. It didn't seem to matter what we tried, what we did, it only seem to be getting worst as the days passed us.

She'd have seizures almost every night after going to bed. There was no rhyme or reason to this, she'd go to bed and within an hour usually she'd wake with treacherous screaming. She wouldn't wake up, she would just scream and scream and scream. We'd try to wake her with no results, I would hold her close to me and pray over her and beg that

God would heal her. I'd cry over her as her eyes would roll into the back of her head and she'd shake uncontrollably.

I remember night after night of calling the doctors and them telling me that there was nothing they could do, nothing more than what we were already doing. I was so beside myself, no one had answers, and no one could tell me what was going on with our precious little girl. Why was this happening?

It was a hard time not only for her, not only for us as parents, but also for our other two daughters who couldn't understand the circumstances and why we couldn't do anything for her. They would be woken by her screaming at night, they'd cry because they couldn't understand what was happening and why we couldn't fix it.

We'd sit with them and pray, we'd try to explain to them that God loved our precious Pumpkin, and for whatever reason this was part of his plan and in time He would heal her body and make her all better.

There were no answers for us as concerned parents, nothing. We felt helpless with no direction other than to pray. So as Christian parents we prayed, and prayed, and well, prayed. We needed answers that the doctors weren't giving us.

We had reached out to so many doctors, and nothing. We went to different clinics, and nothing. So after much prayer and discussion I felt directed to research. I needed to take a step that we hadn't taken before. I would spend months and endless hours researching.

I wanted to know more about the things the doctors did tell us and the things they hadn't told us. I wanted to know what could cause seizures, & what could cause these horrific tantrums that resulted in mom having bloody noses. I wanted to know what was going on in my child's body. I wanted answers, and I was willing to do whatever I had to do to find out what was going on.

There were other families that had problems like ours and that were searching for answers just like we were. They struggled with doctors not having answers, prescriptions being given without really knowing what the problem truly was. It was so frustrating wondering, what could be causing these problems in children that were states apart.

What did they have in common, what was causing these symptoms, what were the answers for our families?

As if it weren't life altering already having our precious little girl going through all this. Now we'd find out things that would turn our world literally upside down and basically into a roller coaster situation. We weren't prepared, we thought we'd have an answer soon and instead it's like we had an eruption of disaster and chaos thrown in our path.

Things that were in pretty much any food you'd find at the grocery store would become our new nightmare! Who would guess that we'd soon be terrified to even walk into a grocery store with our child.

Preservatives, Artificial Dyes, GMOs, this was just the beginning. We had no idea what this would mean for our family. Continuing to research which would lead me to endless nights of praying, crying, and feeling helpless. I had no idea which way to turn, what was I supposed to do with all this new found information, how was this supposed to help our situation. I felt overwhelmed, frustrated, and quite bewildered.

I continued to do some more research, basically research to help me understand the research I had already done. It was overwhelming however it was worth it! It took me a few months, but I got it figured out, well a few tidbits of it that is. I was able to at least explain it to my husband and encourage him to be on board so that we could really help our daughter the way she needed.

We kept journal after journal, documented everything she ate, drank, every bath and body product she used, even down to which cleaners we were using. Then we'd track symptoms, which could be as little as a rash to a devastating as a seizure. After about a month or so we started seeing patterns, with all these things.

With the patterns now aware to us, I was able to do more research and find out the underlying problem. Our daughter has allergies and sensitivities to things we use every single day in our home. These things that are supposed to be "safe" for our bodies, our families, our children and our pets.

Who would imagine that our daughter would have problems with the soaps that are hypoallergenic, natural, and supposed to be made for children. What in the world is happening is all I could think.

However, here's the part you're going to be quite disturbed by, or at least we were. The cleaners, the food, the bath and body products, and basic day to day items we use are hurting us. Now you may not be suffering from rashes, hives, headaches, seizures, etc. However that doesn't mean your body isn't being affected. We really struggled with how these things could be harming our family so badly. Why would companies make these so called safe products knowing that they could hurt our precious children.

There are many companies that make non-toxic, non-hazardous, hypoallergenic products which are not any of these things. These products are not helping us or cleansing us, instead they are filling our bodies with junk, chemicals, and toxins.

Now this is where I will introduce the toxins or as we like to call them the nasties that are in our everyday life. I'll warn you that these big companies want to hide these things from you, they want to make you think that these things are necessary, that they don't harm you, that it's not scientifically proven to cause these affects etc.

However, let me tell you that those who've done the research know what they're talking about. Our family has personally seen the ups and downs to these nasties. I will explain how these affected our daughter and our family, I'll show you the other side to these and how you can expel them from your day to day life.

So let's start off with one of the most common items that make our world well, colorful! Try going a day without consuming it. That is without looking at every single food item, drinks, etc. that you plan to put into your body. You'll find that artificial dyes aren't just in noticeable items like gelatin, soft drinks, and candies. There are colors in so many products that you'd never even imagine.

Did you know for example that in some fruits they inject coloring to brighten the color. Did you know that those yummy blueberry muffins most likely have red #40 in them to make the color better.

This is just the beginning unfortunately. They're used in your day to day products; in fact did you know that they're also used in your bath and body products.

Think about it, would your child prefer a cereal that is bland in color or bright colors? Are you tempted to buy those pickles that just aren't as green or are you drawn to those bright green ones? Many popular candies, drinks, popsicles, puddings, yogurts, gums, boxed mac n' cheeses, baking mixes, pickles, meats, fruits, sauces and chips contain ingredients such as Yellow #5, Blue #1, and Red #40 and unfortunately these are just the top three of the most popular FDA-permitted ones.

Of course that is just the beginning of course, it's not just our food that is limited by artificial dyes, chances are if you take vitamins, use body wash, laundry detergent, cough syrup, brush your teeth, you're coming into contact with artificial dyes daily and quite frequently.

The safety of products containing artificial colors has been a point of debate for decades. These dyes are toxic, can lead to many different emotional disorders, and can harm your family. Still, nine dyes remain on the FDA's approved list for food use in the United States.

A 2007 British study found that children who consumed a mixture of common synthetic dyes displayed hyperactive behavior within an hour of consumption. (These children had not been diagnosed with ADD or ADHD.) The results, published in The Lancet, prompted Britain's Food Standards Agency to encourage manufacturers to find alternatives to food dyes. In July 2010, the European Parliament's mandate that foods and beverages containing food dyes must be labeled as such went into effect for the entire European Union.

Every year, food manufacturers pour 15 million pounds of artificial food dyes into U.S. foods. That amount only factors in eight different varieties, according to the Center for Science in the Public Interest (CSPI).

Here is some insight to how these colors are being used in our day to day products.

Blue #1 aka Brilliant Blue. An unpublished study suggested the possibility that Blue 1 caused kidney tumors in mice. This is added to many Baked goods, beverages, desert powders, candies, cereal, drugs, marshmallows, and other products.

Blue #2 aka Indigo Carmine. Causes a statistically significant incidence of tumors, particularly brain gliomas, in male rats. You'll find this in Colored beverages, candies, pet food, & other food and drugs.

Citrus red #2 it's toxic to rodents at modest levels and caused tumors of the urinary bladder and possibly other organs. You can find this in skins of Florida oranges.

Green #3 aka Fast Green. Caused significant increases in bladder and testes tumors in male rats. You can find this dye in Drugs, personal care products, cosmetic products except in eye area, candies, beverages, ice cream, sorbet, ingested drugs, lipsticks, and externally applied cosmetics.

Red #3 aka Erythrosine. Recognized in 1990 by the FDA as a thyroid carcinogen in animals and is banned in cosmetics and externally applied drugs. However, you can still find it in Sausage casings, oral medication, maraschino cherries, baked goods, and candies.

Red #40 aka Allura Red. This is the most-widely used and consumed dye. It may accelerate the appearance of immune system tumors in mice. It also causes hypersensitivity (allergy-like) reactions in some consumers and might trigger hyperactivity in children. This is by far one of the most popular dyes and for our daughter, it's her biggest trigger! You'll find this dye in many items such as Beverages, bakery goods, dessert powders, candies, cereals, foods, drugs, and cosmetics.

Yellow #5 aka Tartrazine. Yellow 5 causes sometimes-severe hypersensitivity reactions and might trigger hyperactivity and other behavioral effects in children. This is our daughters other big trigger, she gets sever pain in her muscles when she consumes it. You'll find it in Pet foods, numerous bakery goods, beverages, dessert powders, candies, cereals, gelatin desserts, and many other foods, as well as pharmaceuticals and cosmetics.

Yellow #6 aka Sunset Yellow. Caused adrenal tumors in

animals and occasionally causes severe hypersensitivity reactions. You'll find this one in bakery goods, cereals, beverages, dessert powders, candies, gelatin deserts, sausage, cosmetics, and drugs.

In CSPI's summary of studies on food dyes, you can see that some of the most commonly used food dyes may be linked to numerous forms of cancer. CSPI reported:

"The three most widely used dyes, Red 40, Yellow 5, and Yellow 6, are contaminated with known carcinogens ... Another dye, Red 3, has been acknowledged for years by the Food and Drug Administration to be a carcinogen, yet is still in the food supply."

In their 58-page report, "Food Dyes: A Rainbow of Risks," CSPI revealed that nine of the food dyes currently approved for use in the United States are linked to health issues ranging from cancer and hyperactivity to allergy-like reactions -- and these results were from studies conducted by the chemical industry itself.

As CSPI reported

"Almost all the toxicological studies on dyes were commissioned, conducted, and analyzed by the chemical industry and academic consultants. Ideally, dyes (and other regulated chemicals) would be tested by independent researchers.

Furthermore, virtually all the studies tested individual dyes, whereas many foods and diets contain mixtures of dyes (and other ingredients) that might lead to additive or synergistic effects.

In addition to considerations of organ damage, cancer, birth defects, and allergic reactions, mixtures of dyes (and Yellow 5 tested alone) cause hyperactivity and other behavioral problems in some children.

... Because of those toxicological considerations, including carcinogenicity, hypersensitivity reactions, and behavioral effects,

food dyes cannot be considered safe. The FDA should ban food dyes, which serve no purpose other than a cosmetic effect, though quirks in the law make it difficult to do so (the law should be amended to make it no more difficult to ban food coloring than other food additives).

In the meantime, companies voluntarily should replace dyes with safer, natural coloring."

In the U.S., many popular products rely heavily on artificial colors, which of course places pressure on the FDA to both protect the consumer, and avoid making unnecessary regulations based on shaky & "unproven" evidence that could put such companies out of business.

While companies that use artificial colors as subtle ingredients to enhance the appearance of food, they would have to tweak their recipes. Candy and cereal companies would take the hardest blows because they'd have to use real rather than artificial.

The big kicker for me is that people really truly have no idea how bad this stuff really is for you. There are families that are filling their children with unnecessary medications because they think something is wrong with them, however that's not the case. In fact it could be something they're eating that is the true problem.

Most synthetic dyes are petroleum based, think about that for a moment, want to go shove some petroleum jelly in your mouth, or want to put a quart of motor oil in your mouth? Yeah, me neither. Yet most families might as well be and don't have even an idea.

This is just the tip of the iceberg here people, this is not even close to the trauma that we're providing for our children. The FDA doesn't want you to know the truth about these things.

Why? It's because they'd lose money, companies, sales would go down, medical costs would go down and then the pharmaceuticals would lose money as well. It is one big 'ol tangled up mess of business and money, with no concern for the consumer.

Preservatives

Now let's talk about preservatives. Many people will go to the grocery store and look at a package only if they're curious of what's in the product. Many don't even worry about this.

However, if you're one of those people, we know that we can look at just about any product these days and there will be multiple ingredients to which you have no clue what they are, how to pronounce them, and are pretty sure that they are not a food product, right?

Most people don't want to look into it further. They don't want the extra hassle of looking into something healthier, because these days healthier means more expensive, more work, and more hassle. To cut to the chase here, sorry Americans but you've gotten lazy. We truly have gotten lazy.

Our grandparents and great-grandparents had it right. They made their food at home, they had gardens, and they bought meat from a deli that wasn't processed or raised it on their own. They didn't go and buy a box of mac and cheese, they got the ingredients out to make pasta, they melted their own cheese, and they made it from scratch. They didn't go to the store and buy a microwave meal; they made a meal from scratch in their own kitchen with their own hands.

Now a days, homemade means that I pulled it out of a box; I added water and oil and put it in the oven or skillet. That sure is some homemade right there. Now I am pretty sure I'm going to step on some toes here, and well that's okay, because I feel that God is calling me to call you out!

For our family this is not an option, our daughter struggles with pretty much anything processed. A microwave dinner and even most boxed meals result in a horrible rash that will surround her mouth. The picture does no justice for how bad the rashes can get. This was after eating a popular boxed meal. We knew there weren't artificial dyes but hadn't found out yet about our daughter's allergies to preservatives at this time.

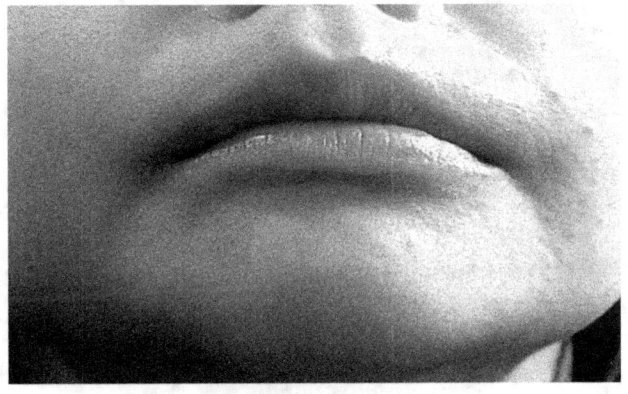

(Notice the rash, it got worse with time)

You'll find the picture below the ingredient list for the boxed meal. Let's take a look shall we, I'll only do a couple otherwise it would take up the entire book.

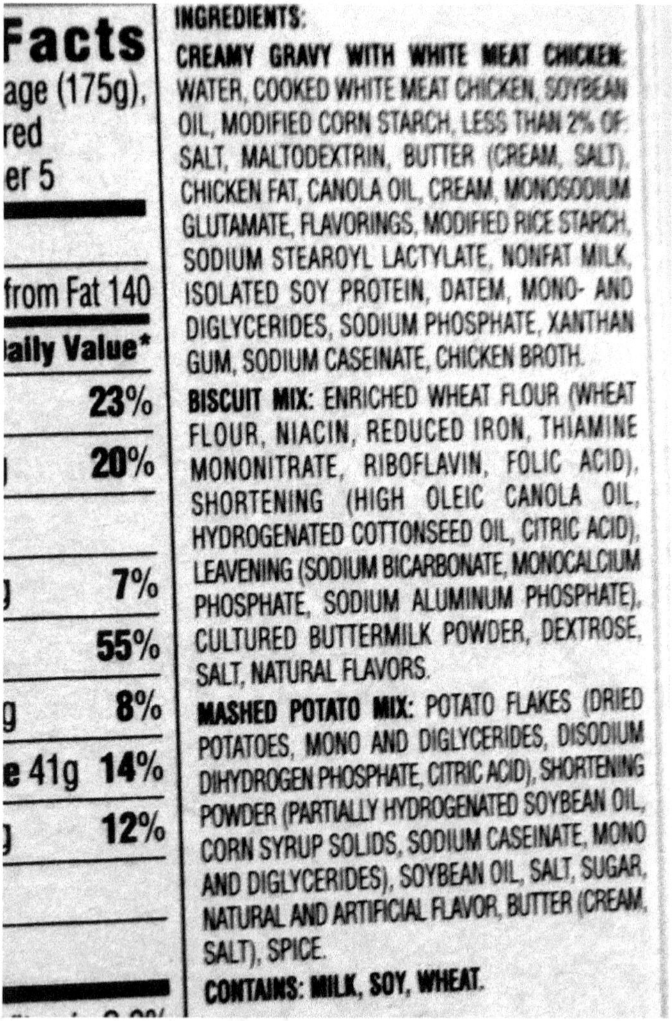

Facts
age (175g),
red
er 5

from Fat 140
aily Value*

	23%
	20%
	7%
	55%
g	8%
e 41g	14%
	12%

INGREDIENTS:

CREAMY GRAVY WITH WHITE MEAT CHICKEN: WATER, COOKED WHITE MEAT CHICKEN, SOYBEAN OIL, MODIFIED CORN STARCH, LESS THAN 2% OF: SALT, MALTODEXTRIN, BUTTER (CREAM, SALT), CHICKEN FAT, CANOLA OIL, CREAM, MONOSODIUM GLUTAMATE, FLAVORINGS, MODIFIED RICE STARCH, SODIUM STEAROYL LACTYLATE, NONFAT MILK, ISOLATED SOY PROTEIN, DATEM, MONO- AND DIGLYCERIDES, SODIUM PHOSPHATE, XANTHAN GUM, SODIUM CASEINATE, CHICKEN BROTH.

BISCUIT MIX: ENRICHED WHEAT FLOUR (WHEAT FLOUR, NIACIN, REDUCED IRON, THIAMINE MONONITRATE, RIBOFLAVIN, FOLIC ACID), SHORTENING (HIGH OLEIC CANOLA OIL, HYDROGENATED COTTONSEED OIL, CITRIC ACID), LEAVENING (SODIUM BICARBONATE, MONOCALCIUM PHOSPHATE, SODIUM ALUMINUM PHOSPHATE), CULTURED BUTTERMILK POWDER, DEXTROSE, SALT, NATURAL FLAVORS.

MASHED POTATO MIX: POTATO FLAKES (DRIED POTATOES, MONO AND DIGLYCERIDES, DISODIUM DIHYDROGEN PHOSPHATE, CITRIC ACID), SHORTENING POWDER (PARTIALLY HYDROGENATED SOYBEAN OIL, CORN SYRUP SOLIDS, SODIUM CASEINATE, MONO AND DIGLYCERIDES), SOYBEAN OIL, SALT, SUGAR, NATURAL AND ARTIFICIAL FLAVOR, BUTTER (CREAM, SALT), SPICE.

CONTAINS: MILK, SOY, WHEAT.

Modified corn starch (GMO), Maltodextrin has a few issues to start off it's an easily absorbed and gets into your bloodstream fast. If there is nothing for all that blood sugar to do (i.e. repair muscle-tissue, give energy), it will get stored as fat. Contrast that with real complex carbs from whole grains, which are broken down and absorbed slowly, and maltodextrin looks more and more like sugar. It has also been associated with Chrohn's disease and to top it off is GMO.

Monosodium glutamate (MSG) a flavor enhancer known to be used in many Chinese dishes has been strewn into thousands of the foods you and your family regularly eat, especially if you are like most Americans and eat the majority of your food as processed foods or in restaurants. MSG is one of the worst food additives on the market and is used in canned soups, crackers, meats, salad dressings, frozen dinners and much more. It's found in your local supermarket and restaurants, in your child's school cafeteria and, amazingly, even in baby food and infant formula.

MSG is more than just a seasoning like salt and pepper, it actually enhances the flavor of foods, making processed meats and frozen dinners taste fresher and smell better, salad dressings more tasty, and canned foods less tinny. While MSG's benefits to the food industry are quite clear, this food additive could be slowly and silently doing major damage to your health.

Many adverse effects have also been linked to regular consumption of MSG, including: Obesity, eye damage, headaches, fatigue and disorientation, & depression. Further, even the FDA admits that "short-term reactions" known as MSG Symptom Complex can occur in certain groups of people, namely those who have eaten "large doses" of MSG or those who have asthma.

According to the FDA, MSG Symptom Complex can involve symptoms such as: Numbness, burning sensation, tingling, facial pressure or tightness, chest pain or difficulty breathing, headache, nausea, rapid heartbeat, drowsiness, weakness. Here is a list of ingredients that ALWAYS contain MSG: Autolyzed yeast, calcium caseinate, gelatin, glutamate, glutamic acid, hydrolyzed protein, monopotassium glutamate, monosodium glutamate, sodium caseinate, textured protein, yeast extract, yeast food, yeast nutrient.

As you can see, with listing only two ingredients from this list, it can become overwhelming and can take charge over you immune system and your child's body as well as yours.

Now you're probably wondering, just why it is that we need all the artificial additives. Well technically we don't, however big time companies like them because they extend shelf life. Man-made preservatives give food and cosmetics a longer shelf life, which allows manufacturers to bring in bigger revenue. Additives are also used to preserve flavor and color.

For centuries people have used salts, vinegar, smoking meats, herbs, boiling and refrigeration to naturally preserve whole food items, but in the last 50 years man-made preservatives have become the common method.

The most popular chemical additives in the food industry today are benzoates, nitrites, sulphites and sorbates. These additives kill and prevent molds and yeast from growing on food. Sulfur dioxide is the most common man-made preservative; it acts as a bleaching agent in food. There are more than 300 additives used today. Did you just read that right?

Yes! There are more than 300 additives used today! Obviously I'm not going to list every single one here or you'd never stop reading, just kidding. However, I will include the link, List of Additives & What They Do by Anne Marie Helmenstine, Ph.D. Chemistry Expert here that includes the extensive list.

So be sure to check out the link I've included here.
http://chemistry.about.com/od/foodcookingchemistry/a/fo
odadditives.htm

Pesticides

As if I haven't already over run your mind with all these additives, let's move on to pesticides. The risks and horrible effects on your health and body are enough reasons to make our family decide to stay as clear and far away from them as possible. You'll find that after reading about them, you'll probably understand and may reconsider what food items you'll be purchasing as well.

Unfortunately, pesticides attack your body in many different ways. Keep this list handy the next time you find yourself wondering if you should buy a carton of conventional strawberries rather than organic to potentially save a few pennies. Remember that all of the following conditions and medical bills will cost you much more than money; the effects of pesticides will cost you your health and maybe even your life or your child's life.

Here are 7 nasty and crazy effects of pesticides that you would have never thought of or even considered. Cancer, Obesity and Diabetes, Parkinson's disease, Infertility, Birth Defects, and Autism. There are many ways to learn more about this and you'll find some resources located in the book to help you grow in understand the things discussed here.

I'd also like to touch base on GMO's "genetically modified organisms" and the truth that is kept from you and your loved ones. So let's start off with what GMO's are. GMOs (or "genetically modified organisms") are living organisms whose genetic material has been artificially manipulated in a laboratory through genetic engineering, or GE. This relatively new science creates unstable combinations of plant, animal, bacterial and viral genes that do not occur in nature or through traditional crossbreeding methods.

Most developed nations do not consider GMOs to be safe. In more than 60 countries around the world, including Australia, Japan, and all of the countries in the European Union, there are significant restrictions or outright bans on the production and sale of GMOs. In the U.S., the government has approved GMOs based on studies conducted by the same corporations that created them and profit from their sale. Increasingly, Americans are taking matters into their own hands and choosing to opt out of the GMO experiment.

Unfortunately GMO products do not have to labeled in the United States. Wonder why this is, well it's because the FDA does not see it as something that is a concern. I will strongly disagree with them as GMO's have been banned in many other countries, yet not in the U.S.

This is the reason that the USDA Organic campaign began, for people and families like ours who don't want GMO's & for the families that want better for themselves. The Non-GMO Project is a non-profit organization with a mission of protecting the Non-GMO food supply and giving consumers an informed choice. If people stop buying GMOs, companies will stop using them and farmers will stop growing them.

Here's some food for thought, in the U.S., GMOs are in as much as 80% of conventional processed food.

So after reviewing the additives and pesticides our government and FDA have approved for us and our families to consume, I'd like to move on and share my views with you.

God did not intend for our bodies to be filled with

artificial, processed crap! Man has decided that it's convenient, it's cheaper to do this way, and it sells!! Maybe that's why America has the largest population of obesity, they blame it on video games, eating too much, sitting around, and not being active enough.

Well now don't get me wrong, I'm not saying that these don't contribute however, I'm married to a farm boy who ate lots, and I'm talking lots. He's got a good healthy appetite like most farm/country boys do.

Here's the difference though, he drank raw milk right from the tank, ate meat that wasn't filled with hormones and other nasty unnecessary chemicals, and he ate plenty of vegetables and fruit right from his loving grandmothers garden.

Notice something here, lack of preservatives, dyes, fillers, and unnecessary products. He ate 100% natural food products that God intended him to have. He is well you could say "as healthy as a horse" for the most part. He didn't have many health problems until his consumption of soda pop and artificial junk made its way into his eating patterns.

When he started consuming these items he started noticing problems with his health. He gained a good sum of weight; he'd have dizzy spells, feel faint at times, and feel queasy if he didn't have something loaded with sugar or something processed.

This is why I'm sharing this information with everyone these things don't just affect our children they affect us as well. Our day to day life, our health, our children's health, and our future generations will be affected, so why not make the change.

As you've read this far you know that these additives and pesticides can make an impact on our lives. For those of you that don't have known sensitivities to them, it may seem like a shock.

However it's not overwhelming or terrifying to the point of saying "yes, we're making the change." However, for our daughter, it is a terrifying and quite overwhelming thing. For our family, it's overwhelming and still to this day takes our breath away.

Just going to the grocery store, is a nightmare for me as her mom. I dread walking down those aisles. Most moms look at the escape from children, some free time, some time to just relax and grocery shop. However, for this mama, it's a completely different story.

I have to go through the aisles knowing that pretty much any item I pick up will have something that will hurt our daughter. It won't matter if it's something she'd love because it is new or because it tastes like strawberries, which she loves. You must look past the cute package and smells and the feeling you get when you read the label and know you won't be able to purchase it. I'm always reminded that it has artificial colors that will cause her to have seizures, if it has preservatives it will cause her to have a horrible rash or hives.

She may enjoy it for a short while, but then she will suffer. She will be in horrible pain and suffering if I give her that small amount of joy from this new item. So I will walk on and keep trying, keep attempting, keep wondering if I'll find anything she'll be able to have without the pain and suffering.

Going to the grocery store, brings me into a state of depression. I find myself suddenly in a rut of which I will struggle with the rest of that day. I will continue to wonder, "why" and think that if they just cared a little more, these companies could change the lives of so many.

Then I will move on, I will be home with my amazing husband and our precious girls and think, nothing will keep

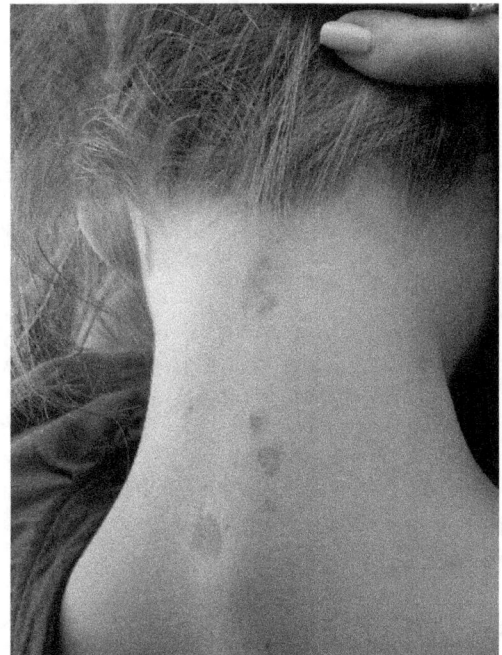

us down. God has this; he always has and always will.
(Pumpkin broke out from allergies to dyes '14)

I'm going to touch on yet another tough bit, something you use every day in your home and don't think twice about. Bath and body products, such as shampoo, conditioner, lotions, makeup, aftershave, shaving creams, bubble bath, and other products you use each day.

You'll find below that I've included many ingredients that are toxic to our bodies. These are things that these large companies don't want you to know about. They will false advertise to sell the product, they will put a fancy cover on, they will say recycled materials, and well blah blah blah and so forth and so on just to sell.

Now for us this is a huge deal because with our daughter she has an extreme sensitivity to scents. If it was made by

God, she is just fine or so it seems at this time. However, if it is artificial in any way, she gets headaches and becomes ill.

In the picture above, it was before we knew she had sensitivities to artificial dyes and fragrances. We had a hard time understanding why it was every time she had a bath she'd break out in a rash. This was hard for us as she did and well still does love bath time.

Now as most of us know, bubble baths, shampoos, and other products that are made for children are usually scented. Why is this, well for the sale of course. Children are taught that if it looks colorful or smells good that it is desirable. Unfortunately it's not just children that are drawn to and desire these things. We all are, I will admit I have to catch myself at times still to this day even though I've been doing this for a couple years now.

For me I can't wear perfumes, lotions, or even makeup that has anything artificial because of our daughter. If she is anywhere near me or she touches my skin with hers, we end up dealing with rashes, hives, headaches, body aches, and more.

Now I've heard "it's all in your head" and even "it's all in her head" let me make this very clear, it's not. Our bodies know what is good for them and what is a toxin.   God created our bodies to know this, for its own protection. The sad part is that our bodies are so full of toxins that once we take them away they don't know what to do. We've provided toxins for so long that our bodies have quit fighting and the disease, illness, and toxins have taken control equaling bad health.

Let's touch base on some harmful ingredients to watch out for:

Alkyl-phenol ethoxylades are used in cleaning products

and shampoos. By mimicking estrogen in the body these are a cause of reproductive cancers and infertility in men and women. Ethoxalades contaminate water.

Benzene, Benzalkonium Chloride, and Benzethonium Chloride is carcinogenic, is not excreted readily and can interact with DNA to produce harmful mutations. It is not normally listed as an ingredient because labeling laws do not require disclosure of trace amounts! Synthetic germicides belonging to the large group of germicides known as "Quats, found in numerous household disinfectants, sanitizers including hand sanitizers and personal care products - long term use may affect immune system, cause asthma and should be especially avoided if you have COPD, or any other form of pulmonary disease.

Colors & Dyes (FD & C or D & C) are predominantly made from coal tar and as such, are carcinogenic, linked to ADD, ADHD and some to thyroid tumors, cause allergies and damage the skin.

DEA (diethanolamine) is a solvent and detergent that is carcinogenic and attacks the liver, kidneys and pancreas. You can find DEA in shampoos, body washes, bubble bath, and shaving cream. It is a health risk to children and babies, linked to miscarriage and harmful to brain development.

Formaldehyde is carcinogenic and breaks down the skin's DNA. It is released by the harmless sounding preservatives DMDM hydantoin or MDM hydantoin, which are common in lotions and soaps. You can also find this in many nail polishes, makes you want to paint your child's nails doesn't it, not!

Parabens are used as preservatives in body products, and are strongly associated with breast cancer tumors.

Para-aminobenzoic acid (PABA) is a chemical found in the folic acid vitamin and also in several foods including grains, eggs, milk, and meat. It is taken by mouth for skin conditions including vitiligo, pemphigus, dermatomyositis, morphea, lymphoblastoma cutis, Peyronie's disease, and scleroderma. PABA is also used to treat infertility in women, arthritis, "tired blood" (anemia), rheumatic fever, constipation, systemic lupus erythematosus (SLE), and headaches. It is also used to darken gray hair, prevent hair loss, make skin look younger, and prevent sunburn. PABA is best known as a sunscreen that is applied to the skin (used topically). PABA doesn't seem to be taken by mouth as often as it used to be, possibly because some people question its safety and effectiveness.

Petrolatum, Vaseline and "Mineral" Oil are linked to breast and other cancers, and banned in the EU.

Propyl / Isopropanol / rubbing alcohol causes mental depression, headaches and is carcinogenic. 1 ounce is a fatal dose. Used to clean new containers, it is rarely listed as an ingredient, but present in trace amounts.

Propylene Glycol carries substances directly into the blood stream, is found in brake and hydraulic fluids, anti-freeze and virtually all baby products, moist/baby wipes, makeup, moisturizers, shampoos and conditioners. Mechanics are advised by the Material Safety Data Sheets to avoid skin contact as it causes liver abnormalities and kidney damage. Can cause dermatitis and irritate the eyes and mucous membranes. My husband being a mechanic, he has started wearing gloves for extra protection. I find this irritating that my husband is not only in danger by lifting a hoist with a vehicle above his head but also by all the chemicals and toxins within them.

Sodium Laurel / Laureth Sulphate or SLS is a mechanical degreaser that has become the major ingredient in most shampoos, bubble baths, shaving foam and liquid soaps. It is carcinogenic, linked to cataracts, denatures proteins and changes genetic material found in cells, breaking the skin's structure. Causes canker sores, so check your toothpaste!

Synthetic perfumes or "fragrances" cause headaches, violent coughing, vomiting, dizziness, skin irritation and rashes according to complains to the FDA. Watch out for synthetic "rose", "jasmine" and "lily of the valley". Synthetic fragrances are carcinogens that contribute to environmental pollution, including the Great Lakes.

Triethanolamine (TEA) causes allergic reactions including eye problems, dryness of hair and skin, and could be toxic if absorbed into the body over a long period of time. These chemicals are already restricted in Europe due to known carcinogenic effects (although still in use in the U.S.) You can find TEA in moisturizers, cosmetics, deodorant, toothpaste, body oils, and washes.

This list could continue to go on, however I don't want to lose you entirely and would like for you to be interested enough to read my next chapter and hopefully my next book if I get that far.

I'd like for you to know that there are many companies that label falsely. Now what I mean by this is that there are plenty of companies these days that will put organic based, all natural, organic, etc. on their products.

This was the reason that the FDA was originally formed, however in my opinion they've slacked and fallen to the standards of which they used to stand for. They don't make companies stand by true accurate standards.

These companies can slide by, because they can put natural on any product that has even one simple natural ingredient in it, as well they can put organic on any product that may have even one simple organic ingredient in it, and so forth and so on.

So that organic body wash you bought, sorry to tell you

but unfortunately it's probably not. It's probably only 10% organic. It's loaded with tons of chemicals that are destroying your body and the "cleaning" of your body.

Other countries have banned these chemicals so why is the U.S. FDA allowing these chemicals to fill our bodies, our children's bodies, our lives, and our food.

We just dealt with this again recently with a product we've loved for the past couple of years only to realize that the product was not indeed 100% organic or natural. It truly was only 70% organic and for our Pumpkin this doesn't work.

I wish this was just a bad dream that we could all wake up from, to think that the United States is supposed to be the place of freedom however, and we're trapped within chemical chaos and control. There is freedom from these things, and by far it won't be easy but it will be worth it.

So please really do your research before buying something just because it says that it is organic or natural doesn't mean it truly is. I've heard this so many times from people, that they went to the store and they got this great lotion or shampoo that is natural only to find out that it is not organic or natural and is full of toxins that are dangerous for them.

This harmful ingredients list is not exhaustive and these ingredients may be found in numerous other personal care products than those listed above. Be sure to check your labels carefully, you'll find a larger scale of ingredients below.

- Acrylate
- acid orange 3
- acrylate copolymers
- amorphous silicates benzyl acetate
- blue 1, 2, and 4
- bromonitrodioxane

- bronopol
- bronopol(2-bromo-2-nitropropane-1, 3-diol)
- butyl benzylphthalate
- butylated hydroxyanisole
- butylated hydroxytoluene
- ceteareth-3
- chlorhexidine
- choleth-24
- chrystalline silica
- coal tar dyes
- DEA
- DEA-Cocamide & Lauramide & Oleamide condensates
- DEA-cocamide/lauramide condensates
- DEA-MEA/Acetame,
- DEA-Sodium lauryl sulfate
- diaminoanisole
- diaminophenol
- Diaminotoluene
- diazolidinyl urea
- Diethanolamide-cocamide
- lauramide &   oleamide condensates
- dioctyl adipate
- disperse blue 1
- disperse yellow 3
- DMDM-Hydantoin
- ethoxylated alcohols
- ethyl alcohol
- fluoride
- formaldehyde
- glutaral

- green 1,2, and 3
- hydroquinone
- imidazolidinyl urea
- lanolin
- laureth's methacrylate copolymers
- metheneamine
- methylene chloride
- morpholine
- nitrophenylenediamine
- nonoxynol
- oleth's padimate-o (octyldimethyl para-amino benzoic acid)
- PEG's (polyethylene glycols)
- polyoxymethyleneurea
- polysorbate 60
- polysorbate 80
- polyvinyl acetate, polyvinyl pyrrolidone
- p-phenylphenylenediamine
- pyrocatechol
- pyroglutamic acid
- quaternium-15
- quaternium-26
- red 4,9,17,19,22,33, and 40
- saccharin
- sodium/hydroxynethylglycinate
- talc
- TEA
- vTEA-Sodium lauryl sulfate
- titanium dioxide
- Yellow 5, 6, and 8.

So as you can see, many of the products we're using are

filled with toxins. These are products that we are told are safe for our families, for our bodies, for our health. However, the truth comes out and it's nothing pretty, in fact it's downright ugly and toxic.

The items that you once thought were safe for your babies, children, animals, for yourself are now going to scare you. I don't mean to scare you or make you doubt. I am sharing this with you to help you turn your lifestyle around and make not only yourself healthier but your family, and maybe even future generations.

So now that you've seen the dark side, how about I take you to the brighter side of things..

Let's move on and put things into perspective, learn about taking the next step and I'll show you the ways to make a difference in your life, how to change the way you eat, clean, and live a healthier, happier life in general.

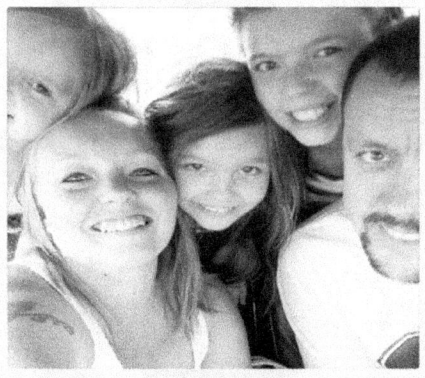

(Our family camping trip 2014)
Sugar 6, Mommy, Pumpkin 8, Sweet Pea 10 & Daddy

But if from there you seek the LORD your God, you will find him if you look for him with all your heart and with all your soul.

-Deuteronomy 4:29

3

PUTTING THINGS INTO PERSPECTIVE,
TAKING THE NEXT STEP

~

"SO WE FIX OUR EYES NOT ON WHAT IS SEEN, BUT
ON WHAT IS UNSEEN. FOR WHAT IS SEEN IS
TEMPORARY, BUT WHAT IS UNSEEN IS ETERNAL."
-2ND CORINTHIANS 4:18 NIV

Let me start off by saying this next part may seem scarier to some than others. Trust me though, it's worth it. This is the part of the journey that changes everything, trust in God and know that he's got this. With him we have no worries!

In the previous chapter I shared with you about the damage that is occurring. The additives, the pesticides, and GMO's. Now I will encourage you, help you along the next part of the journey and help you find the resources to make the change for yourself, your family, or whoever it is that you're helping make this change.

It won't be easy; I won't even begin to sugar coat it. However I will tell you that once you start making the changes and you see the differences you'll be drawn and encouraged to continue to make changes. You'll even find that if you take a step back and stop making the changes that your body will actually rebel. It doesn't want the junk in it; it was not created to handle the junk and the toxins that we've been putting into them for so long.

Now trust me, by no means will this be an easy task, it will keep you on your toes, it will break you down, it will test your patience, it will make you even question your sanity at times. Trust me I know. But it will be worth it that much I can say.

"So do not fear, for I am with you; do not be dismayed, for I am your God. I will strengthen you and help you; I will uphold you with my righteous right hand."
-Isaiah 41:10 (NIV)

This is where we begin, the change, the new perspective, the criticism, the new mark on your life. This is where it all becomes real, this is where you make the choice to trust that God's righteous hand has you near and that you can conquer and challenge.

You can make the changes in your life that everyone has been telling you is just a false hope, and an untrue circumstance, we did. We trusted in God. What does this change mean for you? Will you change your life by eating different, will you heal your body, and will you walk away from obesity, eating disorders or chronic pain?

For our family, making the change meant protecting and healing our daughter first off. Then it suddenly meant changing our lives all together. We're all healthier; we don't follow by what the world tells us, we don't listen to the chaos. We live by the amazing changes and style that God has led us to live by. It meant healing our children, our bodies, and our lives.

We're not doing this lifestyle change to become famous, because quite frankly God knows us and our hearts. He heals us, all we need to do is listen and let Him guide us. For us this means eating differently, making things at home that others would rather just run to the grocery store and buy, it means taking chances of being the outcasts, and above all it means trusting that God will guide and direct us.

Let's begin talking about the things you can do to make the little changes that will make a huge difference in your life and in your health.

Food This is a great place to start. Food is what most of this book revolves around, Organic is by far the best choice for you and your family. This may seem like a long shot for many families, for us it did at first too. To be honest it seems not only scary but unfortunately expensive.

We are a family that lives on one income because God has called my husband and I to agree that my place is to be at home with our daughters. I quit my job and have been at home with our daughters ever since. We homeschool our daughters and had to learn what and how to buy organic.

Now please don't feel discouraged, we can completely relate to the budget part. It's hard to swallow that a gallon of organic milk is $6.00 versus the regular hormone processed milk is only $3.50 or so for a gallon. You'll find that organic does cost more, that's because they can't just toss these items on a shelf and expect it to last a year.

This is where I have to remind myself to keep this bible verse at hand or in mind while I'm grocery shopping.

Psalm 55:2 Hear me and answer me. My thoughts trouble me and I am distraught. (NIV)

Otherwise who knows what kind of trouble I may find myself in. I am a Christian woman, however keep in mind after all I am still human. I'll admit I get downright angry at times still to this day when I go grocery shopping. People probably look at me and think "man that lady is crazy!" I might be, but only a little bit. Because obviously I must be at least a little bit crazy to love life this much and be excited to make my own food at home! Just kidding, I love making my own food at home, I love having the desire to provide better for my family.

I love those random moments when I'm in my kitchen and I'm singing praise music, all while I'm getting all covered in flour and looking like the Pillsbury dough girl. Keep in mind; my three girls are usually included in the pasta making process, so usually this results in four flour covered ladies.

These are the things that I must keep in mind as I stroll through the grocery store these days. Looking forward to teaching my daughters the amazing and underrated glories that the amazing and great women of the past used to do as a necessity. We don't have to do this, we just love doing it as it has become something special for us to share and hopefully one day they will share with their children.

So getting back on track. Food can be a breaking horrible condemning thing to our bodies, or it can be a healing, comforting, real thing that will help us grow and experience life like we've never thought before.

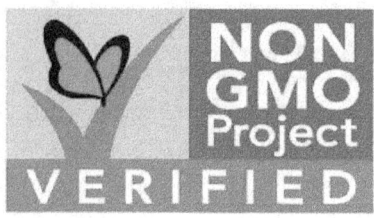

The Non-GMO Project has formed a great service. For those of us who are worried about having non-gmo foods, foods that are covered in pesticides that harm our bodies, and that aren't infused you may say with synthetic dyes this is where we turn. I'd like to explain in a bit more detail here, because quite frankly I LOVE this program and am thankful for it every day of my life.

The Non-GMO Project started in Berkeley, at The Natural Grocery Co., which is a small neighborhood natural grocery store. In 2003, in response to letters from customers who were concerned about a GM soy lecithin that the store was carrying, a group of employees initiated the "People Want to Know Campaign." This effort rallied 161 grocery stores and co-ops throughout the United States in a letter-writing campaign to manufacturers of natural food products and supplements in the U.S. The goal was to discover the GMO status of products, so that the stores' consumers could be offered an informed choice. The results of this campaign were mixed, with a central problem being the lack of a consistent, industry-wide standard for what non-GMO was.

Prior to this, in 2001, The Big Carrot Natural Food Market in Toronto, Ontario implemented a non-GMO purchasing policy after a year and a half of research. They simply discontinued those product lines that were not confirmed by the manufacturer to be non-GMO. It was a radical and very successful move for the store. But the absence of an authoritative standard for non-GMO created problems for this effort, as well, and led The Big Carrot to look for a more comprehensive and reliable way in which to continue providing its customers with non-GMO foods.

In 2005, The Natural Grocery Company and the Big Carrot Natural Food Market teamed up to form the Non-GMO Project, with a common goal of creating a standardized meaning of non-GMO for the North American food industry. To give the Project the rigorous scientific foundation and world-class technical support necessary for this endeavor, the stores began working with the Global ID Group, the world's leaders in non-GMO testing, certification, and consulting.

In the spring of 2007, the Non-GMO Project expanded its Board of Directors to include representatives from all stakeholder groups in the natural products industry, including consumers, retailers, farmers, and manufacturers.

So be sure to check out the resources they offer, they have great answers to questions when you're beginning with organic foods. You'll find resources for companies that are Non-GMO and you can even find the USDA Organic sticker that you'll learn to look for every time you go shopping.

Don't worry though, there are many other ways to buy organic without going to the grocery store. There are these amazing things called Farmers Markets. Not being sarcastic, just seriously for the longest time I had no idea what the heck a farmer's market was. I was totally naive to the concept of these awesome farmers and the Amish/Mennonite community coming together and selling fresh produce.

You can usually look up farmer markets in your local community. For us, living in Wisconsin we usually only see them in the summer and early fall. This makes me sad, because I must admit I love the fresh produce from the local vendors. Do be advised though that you should always look and ask to see if the vendor is indeed organic.

We ask our local vendors these three questions.

1. Do you use pesticides or herbicides?

2. Do you use any sort of artificial preservatives? (More so for baked goods, jam, jelly, etc.)

3. Do you use any artificial colors? (Also more so for baked goods, jam, jelly, etc.)

When we're looking for meats with our local vendors we ask these three questions.

1. What do you feed the animals? (Free range, grass fed, non gmo food products) are what we look for.

2. Do you use hormones?

3. Do you use antibiotics (if only used rarely we are okay with it, however if used regularly we tend to avoid it)

You can always grow your own garden or container garden if space is limited (you can find great resources my facebook page, pinterest page and website).

If you choose to do your own garden, be sure you buy USDA Organic seeds though, unless you've previously bought fresh organic produce, then you can save the seeds and you can plant those.

You'll trash those commercial foods and products in your cupboards and you'll be making your own in the comfort of your own kitchen before too long.

Bath and Body products: This is what we'll hit on next because obviously we all need them right! However they are filled with so much junk that we just don't need.

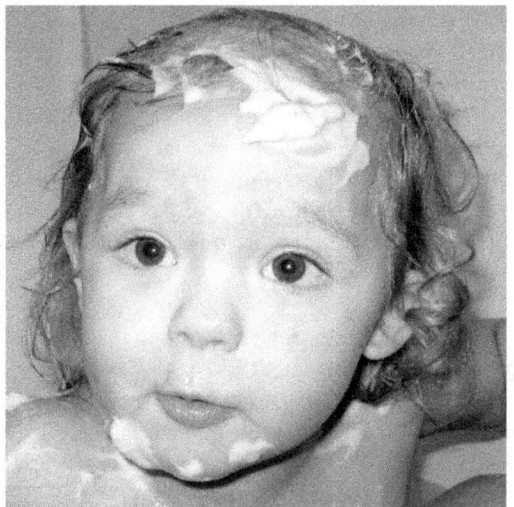

(Here's Pumpkin enjoying a bath, seems like forever ago) Unfortunately after her bath she broke out in a horrible rash!

Remember how we discussed that our food is filled with synthetic dyes, preservatives, and other junk. Well our bath and body products are as well. Just think every time you wash your hair, your child's hair, or wash your body it's being overwhelmed with chemicals, toxins, and junk.

For a long time I could never understand why it was that after we gave our daughters baths the one would always have headaches. We were beside ourselves trying to figure out what in the world was going on. The only time these strange headaches came on was when we gave them baths, or were cleaning the house.

Of course I became frustrated and wanted to know if it was something we were using, we tried different shampoos and conditioners with no results. We tried different bubble bath products, and we even tried different body washes with no results.

I went to the store and saw many products, some that said natural, some that said organic, and some that did not state any of this. I thought natural; yeah that is what I'm looking for. I picked up the bottle and found myself confused; it said natural right on the label. Yet once I started reading the ingredients, or you might say attempted to read them. I couldn't, who the heck can, a chemist maybe but surely not some mama from Wisconsin! I found myself overwhelmed.

I then went down the aisle to the "organic" bottle, thinking yay organic, this won't let me down. What a letdown, as soon as I looked at the ingredient list, I once again was frustrated and overwhelmed. So called organic, do you want to know the truth? Well, you'd better because I'm going to lay it out right here for you.

Just because it says natural or organic does NOT mean that it is. Most of the time (not 100%) companies use false advertisement to get you to buy their product. It is frustrating to many who actually know what they are looking for and it can be overwhelming to those just starting out.

There are plenty of companies that use organic or natural in their names, the way they get by this is because the FDA does not have strict standards for evaluation on cosmetic lines. Let me ask you a question, have you ever seen an unnatural apple or strawberry? Of course not! They are natural; however it doesn't mean that it's organic.

That's how they can get away with it. If there is one natural item in their product they can say, it's natural. If there is one single ingredient, only one in a whole batch of toxic chemicals they can throw organic into the name. How's that make you feel? Me personally, it irritates me and frustrates me, so much to the point that I'd like to write to each and every company that false advertises and give them a piece of my mind.

Now moving on to children's products. Think about all those bottles of bubble bath, baby bath, lotions, etc. Those that we've trusted for so long for those precious little ones whom we care so dearly about. The little miracles that God has blessed us with, that we want to keep safe and protect. We are pouring these horrible chemicals into them, unfortunately you might as well throw them into a toxic pit. Yes it's harsh, but honestly people it's what we've been doing for the past thirty plus years.

We're shoving toxins into our precious babies from the time they're conceived until they leave our home when their eighteen years old. There's a kicker huh? It's not that we want to harm our children in any way, honestly people are doing this blindly, they're led astray by what they think is a good wholesome product for their children.

So this is where the change begins, making a difference for our children, ourselves, our families, our friends, and our world. We take a step in a new direction, now let it be known I promise you that there will be plenty of people who will think this is a bunch of hullabaloo and quite frankly I don't care to waste my time arguing as I've seen the change in our child and am continuing to see changes in our family.

There is always someone to be a critic, but honestly unless they're willing to take a challenge from me and prove me wrong (which obviously will not be happening) I don't care to hear it. My daughter being seizure free for two and a half years and running is plenty enough proof for me. God has led me to write this book and has challenged my whole world and we will make a difference. Even if my book only reaches a few, at least we've made a difference in those few lives.

As if I haven't already overwhelmed you by sharing all this we'll hit our last topic for this chapter, cleaners.

Did you know that accidents are the leading cause of death for Americans between the ages of one and twenty-one, and the fifth leading cause of death for adults. Accidents are the in the home are the second leading cause of accidental death, surpassed only by motor vehicle accidents. In fact many household accidents occur with chemicals, the chemical which we use to clean with.

I'd like to challenge you to look under your kitchen cupboard, bathroom cupboard, in the closet, wherever it is that you keep your cleaning products. Now take a look at them, do you know what half the ingredients are? Can you pronounce them? What's that one? What could it do to a child if swallowed?

Here's a random but very important fact. One ounce, only one small ounce of isopropyl alcohol (rubbing alcohol) can be fatal for your precious child. I'm pretty sure everyone has a bottle of that in their bathroom cupboard or medicine cabinet and hasn't thought twice about it until now. I'll admit, it's in my cupboard and well I'm on the hunt for a natural alternative. We've had a close call with this product, it's clear, it smells horrid (in my opinion) however, to a child that doesn't know what it is, it can become something to play with, drink, or try to play cleaning with.

According to the Environmental Protection Agency (EPA), materials can be classified as hazardous if they are easily ignitable or subject to spontaneous combustion, corrosive, reactive, or toxic.

Before you buy a chemical product, read the label. Can

you feel comfortable having this product in your home with these toxic ingredients? I'd like to share with you some information about the federal ratings for chemicals and how they are based on how hazardous they are to the consumer.

Let's start here:

DANGER: the highest hazard level, the most dangerous product.
WARNING: medium hazard level, a dangerous product.
CAUTION: low hazard level, least toxic.

If the label has no warning, it supposedly means that the product is considered non-hazardous. However in my opinion, if a person of any size can't swallow it without fatal consequences, then it doesn't belong in my home nor is it non-toxic.

Let's move on to the other dark details of chemical cleaners, that you must know to understand why it is we've cut these toxins from our home and why you should as well.

Volatile: Volatile organic compounds (VOC's) are substances that catch fire at a very low temperature (140 degrees Fahrenheit or above) and will be labeled as so: DANGER. HARMFUL OR FATIL IF SWALLOWED. SKIN AND EYE IRRITANT. VAPOR HARMFUL. COMBUSTIBLE.

These materials are called volatile because they evaporate readily, even at very low temperatures; this is why gas stations reek of gasoline even when it is 0 Fahrenheit. A few examples of volatile liquids are petroleum products, paints, kerosene, gasoline, nail polish, and nail polish remover. Obviously we can't get rid of the gasoline, as we need this to run vehicles. However, please if you keep any in a gas can in your garage. Keep the doors locked, keep the cans up so children can't get a hold of these.

Caustic or Corrosive: These strongly acidic or base (alkaline) products will be labeled: DANGER. CORROSIVE. MAY BE ABSORBED THROUGH SKIN. SEVERE RESPITORY AND DIGESTIVE TRACT IRRITANT. MAY CAUSE SKIN AND EYE BURNS.

These products will eat through any organic material they encounter, including your clothing, skin, hair, and eyeballs. Drain cleaners, oven cleaners, toilet bowl cleaners, rust removers, and battery acid are the most common corrosive products in households.

In my personal opinion, if there is a way to avoid these items in my home then I sure will be. I research regularly and this is yet another reason to be writing this book. To share with you how to replace many of these items that have their place in the comfort of our home. After all children are curious, they will investigate and want to explore.

Unfortunately this means that sometimes (especially if homeschooled) they may attempt to experiment with chemicals for science experiments. This is because they're children and they want to explore, experiment, and learn. So for us being a homeschool family, with very curious children; we stay clear of as many of these as possible and recommend the same for other families.

There are many alternatives for these cleaners, I can't wait to share them with you and teach you how to make your own 100% natural cleaners right in the comfort of your own home. Cleaners that your children can help make, and if consumed (which wouldn't be much because they're super bitter/strong/acidic) wouldn't result in fatal results. There's something to put your mind at ease. Oh and those four legged family members won't be harmed by the cleaners either.

This brings me to another thing I'd like to discuss about cleaners and the contamination that they actually produce in the home. When was the last time you thought about the residues from cleaning chemicals and the possible effect they have on you, your family, and your pets?

Residues often build up on surfaces over time, although those residues maybe are hidden by sealers, finishes and everyday soil, grease and grime. One of the issues is that some types of cleaning chemicals are designed to bond with or attract dirt, so their residues continuously compound over and over again. Residues aren't given a lot of attention and, therefore, aren't necessarily considered important.

The point that I'm trying to get across is that these residues are not only on our counters, tables, and other locations in our home. Think about the fact that our food touches these surfaces, our children's sensitive skin comes in contact with these residues and our pets are in contact with these residues as well.

A chemical residue, quite simply, is matter that is left on a surface after evaporation or insufficient rinsing occurs or in this case the residue from the chemicals being used. While you've just cleaned a surface, the particles that adhere to the surface due to residue will provide a food source for microbes feed on. If allowed to grow, those microbes cause the surface to once again become contaminated which then finds their way into your food.

Please also keep in mind that even with laundry detergents you'll find that your clothing actually contains a residue as well. This residue is then in contact with your skin consistently while you're wearing it. This can cause skin rashes, eczema, hives, and skin sensitivity in both children and adults.

You'll really find your next step for all these among the cleaning recipes, which is where the magic begins; well you know what I mean… It's where all the things I've told you start being a part of the past and the new begins for you. You'll learn how to make alternatives that are healthy for you and your family.

You'll learn how to save money and I'm sure if you've got a single cell in your body that craves savings like I do then that's something that has probably caught your attention huh? Well don't worry it will come soon enough, and best of all these great alternatives will not only be healthier for you and your family, but for those adorable furry friends who make their way into your hearts and home. "The other kids".

4

TOXIN OVERLOAD
TIME TO DETOX

~

FOR YOU WERE BOUGHT WITH A PRICE. SO GLORIFY
GOD IN YOUR BODY.
-1 CORINTHIANS 6:20

To those that don't know what it means to detox this is a great place to begin. There are many ways to detox, however some people take it a bit too far. I don't want to guide you into making that mistake, I personally have and it's not a great place to be. Your body rebels and consumes toxins at much a higher rate.

There are many types of detoxes; you'll find horrible recommendations online which I do not in any way agree with. Detox can be quite dangerous if not done correctly. This is why I'd like to share some of my favorites that work great and are safe for both adults and children. Please read all descriptions and information before detoxing.

We hear so much about detoxing cleansing and may wonder just how beneficial it can be. A proper detox or cleansing and good habits for naturally detoxifying the body can really help you to achieve amazing health benefits. The notion of a simple detox program should be integrated into a healthy lifestyle to give you the best results.

Just as you focus on the foods that you eat and proper exercise, there are many other elements to living your best and healthiest lifestyle. Not only do these things factor into detoxifying your body, but there are other simple and highly effective ways to do so as well.

Detoxing is like spring cleaning for our bodies, one traditional method of purifying the body is fasting. However, many people struggle with fasting, nor do they always feel better right away. For some if their liver is not up to par and up for the job, symptoms of toxicity can occur. (I do not recommend for anyone with or has had an eating disorder).

A good 80% of detoxing involves detoxifying potentially harmful substances from our body. Much of this is done by the liver, which is like a clearing house able to recognize millions of potentially harmful chemicals and transform them into something harmless or prepare them for elimination.

Just about any allergic, inflammatory, or metabolic disorder may involve or create optimum liver function, including eczema, asthma, chronic fatigue, chronic arthritis, and hormone imbalances.

If you intend to use a detox to shed pounds, think again. A detox diet isn't indicated for weight loss. In fact, drastically cutting calories can be extremely harmful. When you're not giving yourself a natural amount of calories, fats, carbohydrates and protein, your body's metabolism takes that as a sign that it might not get those things naturally.. It starts to store those things instead of releasing them, so you might find yourself in a worse condition later on. Be wary of any plan that recommends you stop eating in order to cleanse your system.

Take a breather. Deep breathing — especially a technique called ujjayi breathing — may help get rid of toxins in two ways. This technique builds heat in the body so you sweat toxins out and it can help eliminate excess carbon dioxide each time you exhale.

To begin the process, sit in a comfortable position and breathe in and out deeply through your nose. "While inhaling, imagine that your throat is opening as if you were yawning,". "While exhaling, try to constrict the back of the throat and make a soft 'ha' sound as if you're mimicking the sound of the ocean." Silently count to five on each inhale and exhale; continue for five to 15 minutes. Afterward you should feel relaxed and energized.

Snooze to lose. While you're asleep your brain's waste-removal team, called the glymphatic system, is working overtime. Toxic proteins linked to Alzheimer's disease build up while you're awake, getting adequate shut-eye is key to making sure they're cleared out as quickly and efficiently as possible.

Soak in good health. Whether you're really sick or just run-down, chances are you're low on glutathione. Your body naturally makes this protective antioxidant, which zaps free radicals and helps your liver filter out toxins. However, things like stress, illness, and environmental pollution all deplete your levels.

One easy way to build them back up is to take a bath with Epsom salts, which contain sulfur. Sulfur boosts glutathione because glutathione is, in part, made up of sulfur molecules. "Epsom salt also has magnesium, so it will help you relax and sleep." Simply add two cups the next time you draw a hot bath.

Eat clean. Cruciferous veggies such as broccoli, cauliflower, kale, cabbage and bok choy contain phytonutrients that also help your body produce more glutathione. Other detox-friendly foods include dandelion greens, which improve the flow of bile in the liver; celery, which increases urine output; and cilantro, which can help remove heavy metals such as mercury and lead from the body.

Wash down whatever you're munching on with a cup of decaf green tea (I still prefer water though, which is good too) to give your metabolism a kick and further aid in the eradication of unwanted toxins. "If you eat the right foods, the body knows what to do so you can regain your health by eliminating problems such as fatigue, bloating and brain fog."

When you're ready to start your healthy detox, consider making these diet and lifestyle changes: Replace processed foods with whole ones. Do your best to cut out processed foods from your diet, even if you're not ready to cut all of them, cut some little by little.

These include things like store-bought pastries,

microwave dinners, candies — many of the prepared products you find in the middle aisles of your grocery store. Instead of relying on these convenience items, fill up on whole foods such as fruits, vegetables, whole grains, and lean meats and fish.

Increase your fiber intake. Fiber is really important to help the motility in your colon to make sure you're eliminating. If you're detoxing but not eliminating, you're actually creating more problems [in your system}.

There are two kinds of fiber that help promote regularity.

Insoluble fiber, found in leafy greens like spinach and kale, helps keep things moving through your intestines.

Soluble fiber, which comes from foods such as apples, pears and beans, helps bulk up the contents of the bowels. Check out our recipes for ideas on how to include fiber-rich food in your diet.

Increasing your fiber intake means you'll need also need to stay hydrated to keep your bowels moving regularly. Don't go overboard, though — drinking too much water isn't healthy. To determine how much water you need each day, divide your body weight in half and converting that number to ounces. For example, a woman weighing 140 pounds should aim to drink 70 ounces (2 liters) of water each day.

Turn to organic foods when possible, while you don't have to eat only organic, there are certain foods where this is a necessity. The food list known as the "Dirty Dozen" contains a list of foods where pesticides and preservatives can build up and therefore be consumed and ingested by you during digestion.

12 Most Contaminated

Peaches, Apples, Sweet Bell, Peppers, Celery, Nectarines, Strawberries, Cherries, Pears, Grapes (Imported), Spinach, Lettuce, Potatoes.

12 Least Contaminated

Onions, Avocado, Sweet Corn (Frozen), Pineapples, Mango, Asparagus, Sweet Peas(Frozen), Kiwi Fruit, Bananas, Papaya, Cabbage, Broccoli.

You can find more about the the 12 most contaminated and 12 least contaminated at the link listed below.

http://www.organic.org/articles/showarticle/article-214

The rule of thumb generally goes that if you eat the peel or the outside of the fruit or vegetable that you should really opt for organic. Strawberries, apples, and tomatoes are good examples of the types of foods where organic really does matter.

When you choose the right organic foods then you avoid the toxins that can be harmful to your health. This is a simple way of detoxifying the body and all it takes is making good choices at the grocery store.

Drink far more water. Even if you think that you are drinking enough water in a day, take your intake to a whole new level. If there is one thing that can easily and naturally help you to detox your body, it's definitely water. We tend to think that we're drinking enough when we really need to increase our intake dramatically. Water helps flush our body naturally and honestly most of us really don't consume it the way we should. Think about it, we're taught that soda, Kool-

Aid, and other drinks taste better, therefore we tend to resort to these drinks rather than tasteless water.

Water can help to flush out your system naturally, and if you drink enough if it then this happens routinely. Proper water intake can contribute to clearer skin, properly functioning organs, and a more effective circulatory, respiratory, and digestive system. So this one simple substance can offer great help to our entire body and the way that it functions.

Get in more exercise and sweat it out. When you are exercising you are not only helping the body to shed fat and excess weight, but you are also helping to get rid of toxins that may build up. As you sweat these toxins can come out and therefore the cleansing is taking place. Not only that but you are also helping with digestion, circulation, and to keep the organs functioning as they should with a challenging fitness regimen.

The perspiration, the breathing, and the movement all help the body to achieve fitness and also to get rid of the bad and potentially harmful substances that have built up over time.

Probiotics: To be honest, I love probiotics and there are plenty of great ways to introduce them into your lifestyle. You'll also find more about probiotics in the upcoming chapters. Moving on… You may have heard of probiotics or perhaps you don't know much, but these powerful substances help to naturally eliminate bad bacteria in the body.

Probiotics are organisms such as bacteria or yeast that are believed to improve health. They are available in supplements and foods. The idea of taking live bacteria or yeast may seem strange at first. After all, we take antibiotics to fight bacteria. But our bodies naturally teem with such organisms.

The digestive system is home to more than 500 different types of bacteria. They help keep the intestines healthy and assist in digesting food. They are also believed to help the immune system.

Researchers believe that some digestive disorders happen when the balance of friendly bacteria in the intestines becomes disturbed. This can happen after an infection or after taking antibiotics. Intestinal problems can also arise when the lining of the intestines is damaged. Taking probiotics may help.

"Probiotics can improve intestinal function and maintain the integrity of the lining of the intestines," says Stefano Guandalini, MD, professor of pediatrics and gastroenterology at the University of Chicago Medical Center. These friendly organisms may also help fight bacteria that cause diarrhea.

Now you are probably wondering where to find probiotics, this is where I get excited. I like sharing with people the amazing benefits of probiotics and how you can make them a huge part of your daily regimen. Some people here probiotics and think yogurt or pills. However that is just the beginning.

There are many ways of introducing probiotics into your diet, you can make your own recipes at home that will help you supply your family with natural organic probiotics.

Some examples you can make or find quite easily are:

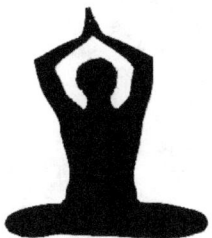

Kefirs, buttermilk, fermented foods, sour dough breads, Kombucha, and even others.

Try yoga for a new type of exercise and meditation. For fellow Christians, there are options for Christians that you can use. We already know that exercise is good for our health and for our ability to cleanse naturally.

Taking it one step further, yoga can be one of the most helpful types of exercise out there when it comes to the body's natural ability to cleanse and get rid of toxins that have built up over time.

These flexibility and balance type of movements can be instrumental to your ability to breath in good cleansing oxygen and breathe out harmful substances within the body. You are getting deep down into muscle tissue as you would with a massage, and you are also helping to breathe out toxins that have built up in your system over time.

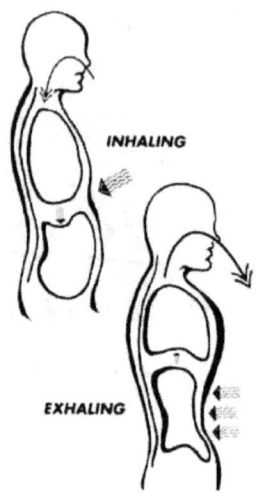

Incorporate super foods into each meal. The great thing about super foods is that they contain important nutrients and antioxidants which our bodies need to fight off infections. The presence of these antioxidants and nutrients in the body help to fight off harmful toxins and substances that may compromise our immune system and our overall health—so the inclusion of them in our diets is critical.

Super foods are a delicious and nutritious group of foods including foods rich in Omega 3 fatty acids; these are just at the top of the list to get you started. Such as: Beans, blueberries, broccoli, oats, oranges, pumpkin, wild salmon (preferably not farm raised), spinach, tomatoes, turkey, walnuts, and yogurt.

Home remedies rather than antibiotics. The very medications that are intended to help your illnesses or health conditions may be contributing to toxins in the body. Though antibiotics and other medications are intended to help you to stay healthy, they also contain harmful substances that can build up in your intestines and digestive system over time.

Though some medications may be very necessary, it's always best to try home remedies whenever possible. If you can fight off a common illness using options like ginger, garlic, essential oils, or other natural herbs or plants, then you have a good chance at achieving better health and performing a cleanse in the process.

Natural home remedies help to get rid of the illness in the way that your body requires. So as they are fighting off the substances or viruses that are making you sick, you are also getting rid of all other harmful toxins in the body. In the "Old days" these were what our grandparents and great grandparents depended on. They didn't turn to medicine, they turned to their gardens and their kitchens for the ailment of which they were dealing with for a natural home remedy.

For us this is what we do, if the signs of a cold are coming on we hit our home remedies and we kick it right from the start. If someone has an ailment which is something we can heal at home, we do it. We don't need to run to the doctor's office at the slightest onset of a cold, chills, fever, or little things anymore. You can find more information about this on my blog, on the facebook page and in my next book as well.

Eliminate daily medication wherever possible. The more you can turn to natural remedies and alternatives the better of you'll be. A truly healthy lifestyle consists of eating the right foods, exercising regularly and challenging yourself, getting plenty of rest, learning to manage your stress, getting rid of the bad habits, performing a regular cleanse, and adapting to a positive and healthy mindset.

If you have medication that is lifesaving then that's a must to continue on with. If however you take medication that could be replaced by natural and healthy home remedies and methods, then that's another way to cleanse and to opt for better and healthier living. Getting rid of any substances that can be construed as toxins by the body, such as regular medications, is always a wise idea.

Turn to natural herbs, homeopathics and holistic medicine. You can turn to homeopathic & holistic medicine and find a whole new world of herbs and natural remedies to help whatever ails you. Some herbs are easy enough to incorporate into your daily life as they are readily available. Options garlic, basil, and even cilantro have some natural cleansing properties and you can easily add them into your favorite dishes or enjoy them on their own. Using these natural herbs can offer great help with cleansing the body, but you do have to be sure to choose which ones are right for you and then use them properly. You may even see some of the results of that happening rather quickly, so don't be alarmed if that happens.

To learn more about natural herbs and holistic medicine, make sure check out the available resources I've listed, check out my blog, fb, pinterest as well as watching for my next book. This is where we'll discuss how natural herbs and holistic medicine can really make a difference in your life.

Juicing. As with anything else, be sure to take your time with this and never go to extremes. Try a new juice 1-2 times a week just to get used to it and to find what works best for you. Then continue to add on until juicing becomes part of your everyday life. A bit of experimenting can ensure that you get some wonderful health benefits and that you learn how to cleanse in the most effective way possible.

Juicing extracts the juice from fresh fruits or vegetables. The resulting liquid contains most of the vitamins, minerals and plant chemicals (phytonutrients) found in the whole fruit. However, whole fruits and vegetables also have healthy fiber, which is lost during most juicing.

Some juicing proponents say that juicing is better for you than is eating whole fruits and vegetables because your body can absorb the nutrients better and it gives your digestive system a rest from working on fiber. They say that juicing can reduce your risk of cancer, boost your immune system, help you remove toxins from your body, and aid in digestion. You want to try to eat whole vegetables too, so try to sneak them in there.

On the other hand, if you don't enjoy eating fresh fruits and vegetables, juicing may be a fun way to add them to your diet or to try fruits and vegetables you normally wouldn't eat. That's the great part of juicing. I personally have a really hard time eating vegetables, so this is a great way for me to get my veggies in.

If you do try juicing, make only as much juice as you can drink at one time because fresh squeezed juice can quickly develop harmful bacteria. And when juicing, try to keep some of the pulp. Not only does it have healthy fiber, but it can help fill you up.

Detox dandelion tea: According to classical homeopathic practitioner Sonya McLeod, B.A., D.C.H., dandelions are a great source of vitamin A, potassium, iron and calcium. According to McLeod, dandelion detox tea is a diuretic that will eliminate bodily toxins through your liver and kidneys. She recommends brewing 6 tablespoons of 1-year-old dried dandelion root and 12 tablespoons of fresh dandelion leaves in 4 cups of purified, boiling water. Other recipes call for simply adding 2 teaspoons of crushed dandelion leaves to a cup of boiling water and allowing it to brew for about 10 minutes.

Oil Pulling: Now some people freak out about this as soon as they hear what it is, some just get grossed out, and some are intrigued and just can't wait to try it. So here we go, onto the glorious details of something so simple that makes such a huge difference.

Oil pulling or oil swishing is a folk remedy where oil is "swished" (kavala graha) or "held" (snigda gandoosha) in the mouth. Practitioners of oil pulling claim it is capable of improving oral and systemic health, including a benefit in conditions such as headaches, migraines, diabetes mellitus, asthma, and acne, as well as whitening teeth. Its promoters claim it works by pulling out "toxins", which are known as ama in Ayurvedic medicine, and thereby reducing inflammation.

Oil pulling therapy can be done using oils like sunflower oil or sesame oil. The sesame plant (Sesamum indicum) of the Pedaliaceae family has been considered a gift of nature to mankind for its nutritional qualities and desirable health effects. Sesame oil is considered to be the queen of oil seed crops because of its beneficiary effects.

*** If you decide to try oil pulling, it is advised not to spit the substance down the drain or into your toilet.

To Oil Pull:

1. Make sure to oil pull first thing when waking, before eating or drinking anything.
2. Swish about 1-2 Tbsp. of organic coconut oil (or organic oil discussed above) your choice with flavor. I prefer coconut, the flavor is very mild and easier to tolerate. You'll swish the oil for 10-20 minutes. (Some people can only tolerate 5, that's okay to start out with, work your way up to the full time).
3. Spit out the oil (into a plastic baggy and throw into the trash, you'll notice that the substance will be a cloudy white looking liquid when you're done) , and rinse. For an extra clean feel, rinse with salt water.
4. Brush your teeth as normal.
5. Repeat this 3-4 times per week for best results.

Detox Baths: A detox bath is one of the easiest healing therapies we can do to facilitate our body's natural detoxification system.

Detoxification of your body through bathing is an ancient remedy that anyone can perform in the comfort of their own home. A detox bath is thought to assist your body in eliminating toxins as well as absorbing the minerals and nutrients that are in the water. Most of all, it'll leave you feeling refreshed and awakened.

Typically, a detox bath is made with Epsom salt also known as magnesium sulfate, which not only draws out toxins, but has health benefits of its own:

- Ease stress and improves sleep and concentration
- Help muscles and nerves function properly
- Regulate activity of 325+ enzymes
- Help prevent artery hardening and blood clots
- Make insulin more effective
- Reduce inflammation to relieve pain and muscle cramps
- Improve oxygen use
- Flush toxins
- Improve absorption of nutrients
- Help form joint proteins, brain tissue and mucin proteins
- Help prevent or ease migraine headaches

1. Prepare your bath on a day that you have at least 40 minutes available. The first 20 minutes are said to help your body remove the toxins, while the second 20 minutes are for absorbing the minerals in the water.

2. Fill your tub with comfortably hot water. Use a chlorine filter if possible.

3. Add Epsom salts (aka magnesium sulfate). Soaking in Epsom salts actually helps replenish the body

magnesium level, combating hypertension. The sulfate flushes toxins and helps form proteins in brain tissue and joints. Epsom salt is very inexpensive. It can be purchased in decently sized bags or cartons at discount stores in the garden center or pharmaceutical area. Very large bags can be ordered from garden centers.

- **For children less than 60 lbs., add 1/2 cup to a standard bath.**
- **For children 60 lbs. to 100 lbs., add 1 cup to a standard bath.**
- **For people 100 lbs. and up, add 2 cups or more to a standard bath.**

1. Add 1 cup of baking soda (a.k.a. sodium bicarbonate). Baking soda is known for its cleansing ability and even has anti-fungal properties. It also leaves skin very soft. Large bags can usually be found in the swimming pool chemical area, but the boxes from the bakery aisle will work fine. (I like to get a nice bulk sized bag from Sam's Club)

Optional, add ground ginger or fresh ginger tea. While this step is optional, ginger can increase your heat levels, helping to sweat out toxins. However, since it is heating to the body, it may cause your skin to turn slightly red for a few minutes, so be careful with the amount you add. (I don't recommend using ginger for children) Depending on the capacity of your tub as well your sensitivity, anywhere from 1 to 3 Tbsp. can be added.

** Most people sweat profusely with the addition of the ginger, and if you wrap your body in a blanket immediately after getting out of the tub, you can continue to detoxify through perspiration for another couple of hours. This is especially beneficial if you are trying to get rid the body of a bug of some sort of disease, like the flu, or a cold.

2. Add aromatherapy oils (please don't use synthetic oils, use a good brand. I prefer organic oils). Again optional, but many people love the fragrance of such oils and for many, the oils have particular therapeutic properties to take advantage of. There are many oils that will make the bath an even more pleasant and relaxing experience (such as lavender and ylang ylang), as well as those that will assist in the detoxification process (tea tree oil or eucalyptus). A couple drops will do just fine. Please read more about essential oils on my blog.

    ** If you prefer, you can use fresh herbs. Add mint leaves (warming), lavender flowers (soothing), chamomile (soothing), or anything else that suits your mood.

3. Swish all of the ingredients around in the tub, and then soak. Again, 40 minutes is recommended (the longer the better), but aim for at least 20. You should start sweating within the first few minutes. If you feel too hot, start adding cold water into the tub until you cool off.

4. Get out of the tub slowly and carefully. Your body has been working hard and you may get lightheaded or feel weak and drained. On top of that, the salts make your tub slippery, so stand with care.

5. Drink plenty of water. Any time your body detoxes (after this type of bath, a massage, or chiropractic work; for example), you need to flush out toxins. If you don't, you will likely feel sick afterwards.

    6. After the bath, you might like to rub down your body with a loofah or vegetable bristle brush. This can help to stimulate the lymphatic system, which can aid with the release of toxins. Use long, gentle sweeping strokes aimed toward the heart.

Some great tips to help you increase the benefits of

your detox bath.

- Play some soothing and interesting music to keep your mind in a relaxed state.
- Relax for the rest of the day and allow your body to continue to detoxify and heal itself.
- Dry brush your entire body before the bath as it gets rid of dead skin cells. It is also beneficial because it helps with circulation of blood and lymph. Lymph is basically your body's garbage system and if you get it circulating before the detox bath, it is very beneficial in helping get rid of additional toxins that may not be sweated out!
- Eucalyptus essential oil in a warm bath helps open breathing passages. (don't overdo it, only use one or two drops)

1. Have your towel nearby the tub and ready so that you can wrap up immediately and continue the detox.
2. Don't eat immediately before or after the bath.
3. It's also a good idea to drink water before and during your bath, especially if you're feeling overheated from the tub water.
4. Don't let your hair in this water the salt will strip it making it feel like hay.
5. Turn off the lights. Light candles. Clear your mind, meditate & relax.
6. Use a deep conditioning treatment on your hair and wrap it up under a cap or towel while you're in the bath.
7. Detox bath should not be done daily.
8. If you are pregnant or have a health condition then consult a doctor

Here are a couple other great Detox Bath ideas.

Bentonite Clay Detox Bath- Bentonite clay is presented as a way of taking a heavy metal detox bath since it is said that it draws these metals out through its magnetism. Heavy metals can enter the body through any number of ways, and chances are if you haven't cleansed your body of them yet, you have accumulated them over the years. The most common way is just by drinking water than hasn't been properly filtered. Other ways are through dental work, eating foods that have been treated with certain chemicals, and much more. That's why it's important to do a regular detox for these heavy metals.

Apple Cider Vinegar Detox Bath- If you're not familiar with the benefits of apple cider vinegar, it's important to take the time to learn about what it can do for you, both taken internally, and used externally to treat a number of conditions. Here they're using it in a detox bath to help with conditions like arthritis and gout, as well as anything else caused by inflammation. This is a good bath to take if you feel you need to sweat the toxins out, and also if you want to make sure that you get to sleep without lying awake with a wandering mind.

Warnings!!!

❖ **Before adding herbs not on the list to your bath, please read what their effects are. Some herbs <u>CAN be poisonous</u>.**

❖ **Do not take a hot bath or a detox bath if you are pregnant, or have heart, kidney, or any other health issues.**

❖ **Avoid putting hydrogen peroxide in your bath. As an oxidizing agent, it can have corrosive effects on your skin.**

❖ **As with any application of essential oils, be aware of the properties of the oils and any** contra-indications (things that might bring about harm) for your particular conditions.

Please advise, really research any detox remedies you may find online!!! Some can be very DANGEROUS!

5

PUTTING "CLEAN"
BACK INTO CLEANING

~

"CREATE IN ME A CLEAN HEART, O GOD, AND
RENEW A RIGHT SPIRIT WITHIN ME."
-PSALM 51:10

This is the last chapter, you've made it through the book. Take a moment and pat yourself on the back, it's truly a tough thing to make it through chapter two. That's where the lack of pizzazz was right?!

Now it's time to give you some quick and simple safe alternatives until my next book comes out. By the way you should really like the next one, especially if you like to cook and make your own stuff. It will be all about making your own healthy alternatives to a LOT of different items that you use every single day.

I make my own cleaners, lotions, body wash, hair products, deodorant, perfume/body spray, laundry detergent etc. You'll find here that I'm going to share just my absolute favorite cleaners. You can also check out my pinterest, blog, and fb page to find more recipes.

Dishwasher Detergent Laundry Soap
*   1 cup washing soda1 cup borax
*   1 cup baking soda1 bar soap flakes
1.   Grate 1 bar of castile soap into flakes.
2.   Mix with the rest of the ingredients.
3.   2 Tbsp. per load Medium or 3 Large for heavier soil, add an additional Tbsp.

Easy Peazy Hardwood Floor Cleaner
*   1/2 cup white vinegar
*   1 gallon warm/hot water.
1.   Wash hardwood floors with white vinegar and water.
2.   Vinegar removes residue built up from other cleaners that attract dirt and grime.

Glass Cleaner
*   ¼ cup vinegar
*   Enough water to fill a one quart spray bottle once vinegar has been added.
1.   Mix and spray.
2.   Spray and Dry with newspaper.

Citrus Disinfectant
- Peels from orange, grapefruit, lemon, or lime
- 3 cups white vinegar
- 1 clean quart jar with lid
- 1 clean 32 oz. spray bottle
1. Combine citrus peel & vinegar in the quart jar.
2. Fasten the lid on the jar and store the mixture in a cupboard for two weeks, giving it a shake occasionally.
3. Once the time has lapsed, strain liquid out. Use for cleaning as directed. ½ citrus solution mixed with ½ water.

Multipurpose Cleaner
- 3 ½ cups hot water
- ½ cup white or apple cider vinegar
- 1 tsp. borax
- 1 tsp. washing soda
- 1 tsp. liquid castile soap
- 1 clean 32 oz. spray bottle
1. Fill spray bottle first with hot water;
then add vinegar, borax, washing soda, and liquid castile soap.
2. Shake well before using.
   Spray and wipe down with a clean cloth.

Herbal Carpet Freshener
- ½ cup lavender flowers
- 1 cup baking soda
1. Crush lavender flowers, mix with b. soda
2. Sprinkle on floor, wait 30 mins. Vacuum.

Pie Spice Room Freshener
- 3 cups water
- 6 cloves1 cinnamon stick
- 6 pieces dried orange peel
1. In small saucepan, combine and bring to boil over med heat.
2. Reduce and simmer, uncovered.
3. Don't let water boil away.

Lemon Oil Furniture Polish
- 1 cup olive oil
- 1/3 cup lemon juice
- 1 clean 16 oz. spray bottle
1. Combine oil and lemon juice in spray bottle.
2. Shake well before using.
3. Apply a small amount to soft cloth and apply evenly over wood surface.
4. Use a clean, dry cloth to buff and polish.

Spot Mold & Mildew Remover
- 1 cup white vinegar
- 2 Tbsp. borax
- 4 cups hot water
- 1 clean 32-oz spray bottle
1. Combine ingredients in the spray bottle & shake to mix.
2. Spray on surface, wipe off with dry cloth.

Nontoxic Rust Remover
- 1 lime (a second may be needed for some jobs
- ¼ cup salt
1. Squeeze the lime over the rust spot, and then cover the moistened area with salt.
2. Let sit for 3-4 hours.
3. Use nylon scrubber to scrub the mixture off.

Nontoxic Toilet Bowl Cleaner
- 1 cup borax
- ½ cup vinegar
1. Flush the toilet to wet the sides of bowl.
2. Sprinkle the borax around the bowl;
3. Then liberally drizzle some vinegar over the top.
4. Let the toilet sit undisturbed for 3 to 4 hours before scrubbing with toilet brush.

Tough Toilet Bowl Cleaner
- 2/3 cup borax
- 1/3 cup lemon juice
1. Combine ingredients to form a paste.
2. Apply the paste to the toilet bowl using a sponge or rag.
3. Let the paste set for 2 hours, then scrub off.
4. Flush toilet.

Drain Opener
- ½ cup baking soda
- 1 cup vinegar
- 1 teapot boiling water
1. Pour baking soda down drain, and then pour in the vinegar.
2. Keep the drain covered for 10 mins, and then flush it out with boiling water.

ABOUT THE AUTHOR

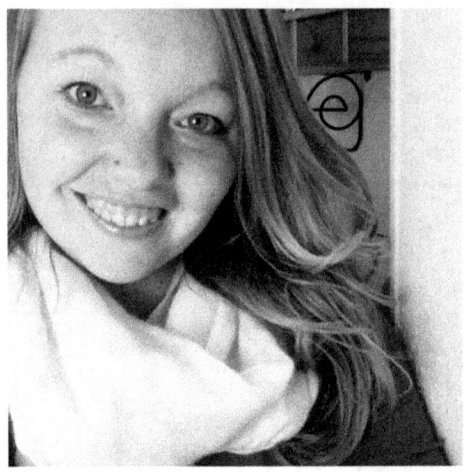

Donna is a small town Wisconsin God love'n gal; she's a smitten wife of over ten years, and homeschooling mom to three girls {listed by their nicknames}.

She adores spending time with her family, friends, and blogging on Beautifully Unprocessed. Donna enjoys cast iron cooking, spending lots of time outdoors, exploring what the world has to offer and finding new ways to live more unaltered.

To learn more or to connect with Donna be sure to check out her blog {resources galore}.

Would you like to know more about starting a relationship with God? Donna would be overjoyed to tell you more and share her story of faith with you.

God bless

NOTES

- Rachel Hennessey Forbes Staff, Living in Color: The Potential Dangers of Artificial Dyes 8/27/2012, http://www.forbes.com/sites /rachelhennessey/ 2012/08/27/living-in-color-the-potential-dangers-of-artificial-dyes/
- The Hidden Health Risks of Food Dyes, By Milton Stokes, M.P.H., R.D., "Live or Let Dye," November/December 2010 http://www.eatingwell.com/ food_ news_origins/food_news/the_hidden_health_risks_of_food_dyes
- Are You or Your Family Eating Toxic Food Dyes? http://articles.mercola.com/sites/articles/archive/2011/02/24/are-you-or-your-family-eating-toxic-food-dyes.aspx
- Center for Science in the Public Interest, Summary of Studies on Food Dyes, (PDF) http://cspinet.org/new/pdf/dyes-problem-table.pdf
- Center for Science in the Public Interest, http://www.cspinet.org/new/ 201006291.html
- Center for Science in the Public Interest, Food Dyes: A Rainbow of Risks (PDF) , http://cspinet.org/new/pdf/food-dyes-rainbow-of-risks.pdf
- Is Maltodextrin Bad for You? The Good, the Bad, & the Ugly, http://fitnessfortravel.com/is-maltodextrin-bad-for-you/
- http://articles.mercola.com/sites/articles/archive/2007/08/28/dangers-of-msg.aspx
- MSG: Is This Silent Killer Lurking in Your Kitchen Cabinets, By Dr. Mercola, http://articles.mercola.com/sites/articles/archive/2009/04/21/msg-is-this-silent-killer-lurking-in-your-kitchen-cabinets.aspx
- FDA Consumer Magazine "MSG: A Common Flavor Enhancer" January-February 2003
- MSG: Is This Silent Killer Lurking in Your Kitchen Cabinets,http://articles.mercola.com/sites/articles/archive/2009/04/21/msg-is-this-silent-killer-lurking-in-your-kitchen-cabinets.aspx
- Dangers of Food Additives, by the editors of PureHealthMD, http://health.howstuffworks.com/wellness/food-nutrition/facts/dangers-of-food-additives.htm
- Center for Science in the Public Interest. (2004). CSPI's guide to food additives'. Center for Science in the Public Interest.
- Karen Lau, W., McLean, G., Williams, D., Howard, C. (2006). Synergistic interactions between commonly used food additives in a developmental neurotoxicity test. Toxicological Sciences,

90(1):178-187.
- http://chemistry.about.com/od/foodcookingchemistry/a/foodadd itives.htm
- 7 Nasty and Crazy Effects of Pesticides in Food, Exposure, http://www.nationofchange.org/7-nasty-and-crazy-effects-pesticides-food-exposure-1350220273
- What is GMO?, Agricultural Crops That Have a Risk of Being GMO, http://www.nongmoproject.org/learn-more/what-is-gmo/
- GMO Facts, Frequently Asked Questions, http://www.nongmoproject.org/learn-more/
- Dangerous Ingredients in Bath & Body Products, by Head Health Nutter , http://livelighter.org/dangerous-ingredients-in-bath-body-products/, By Tracey Tief, Certified Natural Health Practitioner
- http://www.nontoxicalternatives.com/harmful-ingredients-list.html
- CC Medical Devices, Inc, , http://www.arneu.com/TopicalPainReliefCream/page.php?page=t ea
- Harmful Ingredients List,http://www.nontoxicalternatives.com/harmful-ingredients-list.html
- Holy Bible, New International Version®, NIV® Copyright © 1973, 1978, 1984, 2011
- History of The Non-GMO Project, 2014 Non-GMO Project , http://www.nongmoproject.org/
- Organic Housekeeping, Ellen Sandbeck, 2006, pg 300
- Organic Housekeeping, Ellen Sandbeck, 2006, pg301-302
- The Hidden Hazards Of Cleaning Residues By Sam Cooper, January 03, 2013, http://www.cmmonline.com/articles/230092-the-hidden-hazards-of-cleaning-residues
- 28 Simple & Natural Ways to Detox your Body, http://bembu.com/natural-ways-to-detox-your-body
- How to do a healthy detox, By Jennifer Goldberg, http://www.besthealthmag.ca/get-healthy/health/how-to-do-a-healthy-detox